JOSETTE MILGRAM

FACE & BODY

marie claire

MURDOCH BOOKS

face & body

visage et corps
[vizaʒ e kɔʀ]

表面及びボディ

viso e corpo

cara y cuerpo

Gesicht und Körper

面孔和身體

сторона и тело

Contents

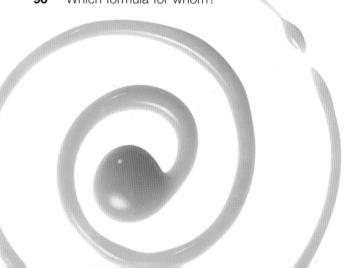

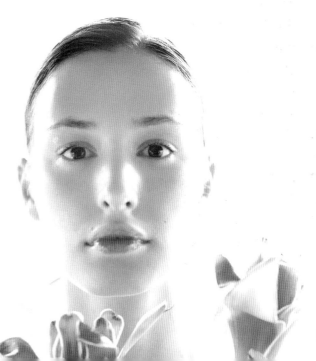

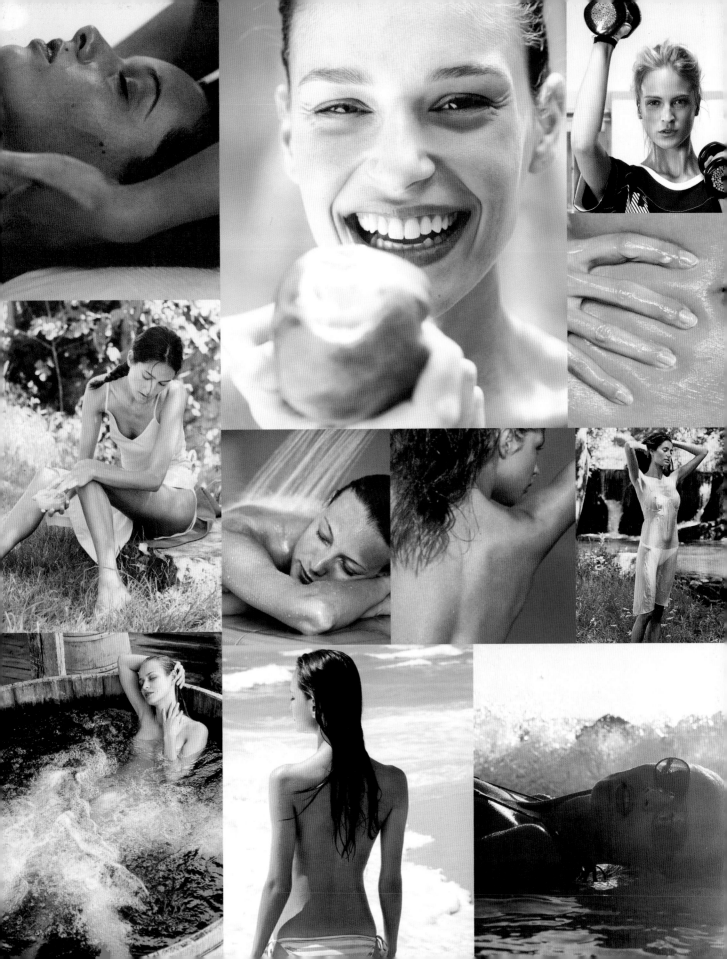

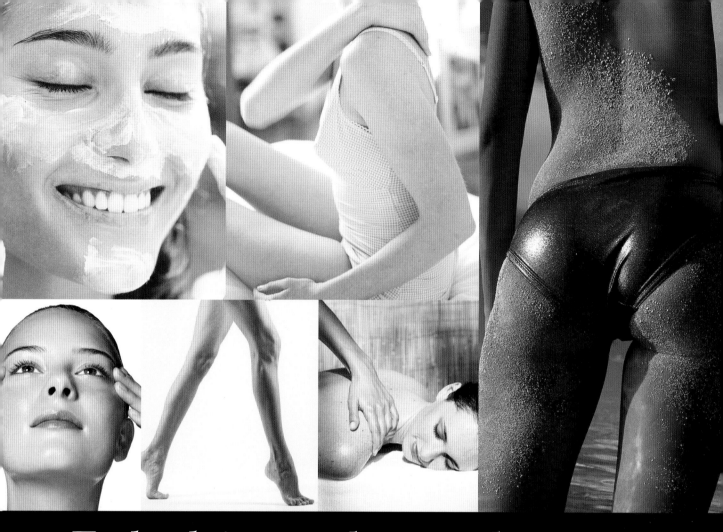

Embodying my beauty dreams…

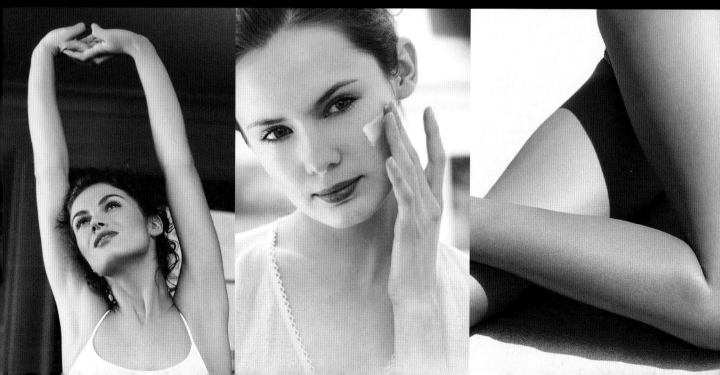

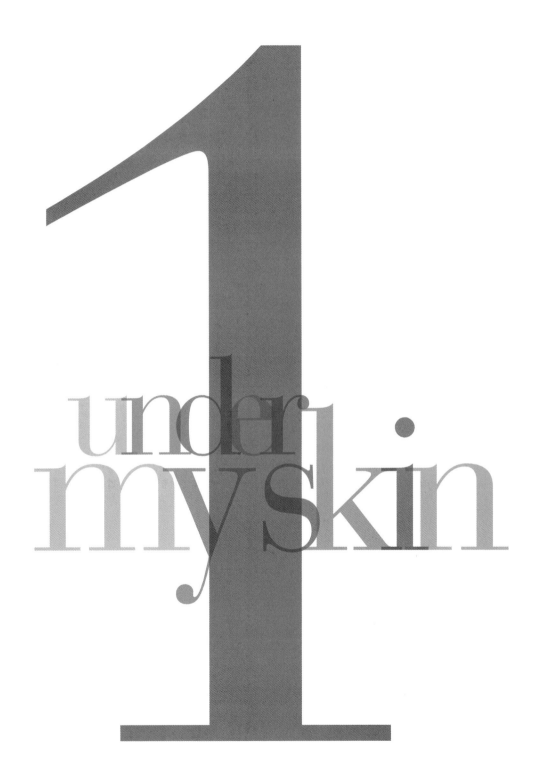

1

under my skin

MY BEAUTY CAPITAL

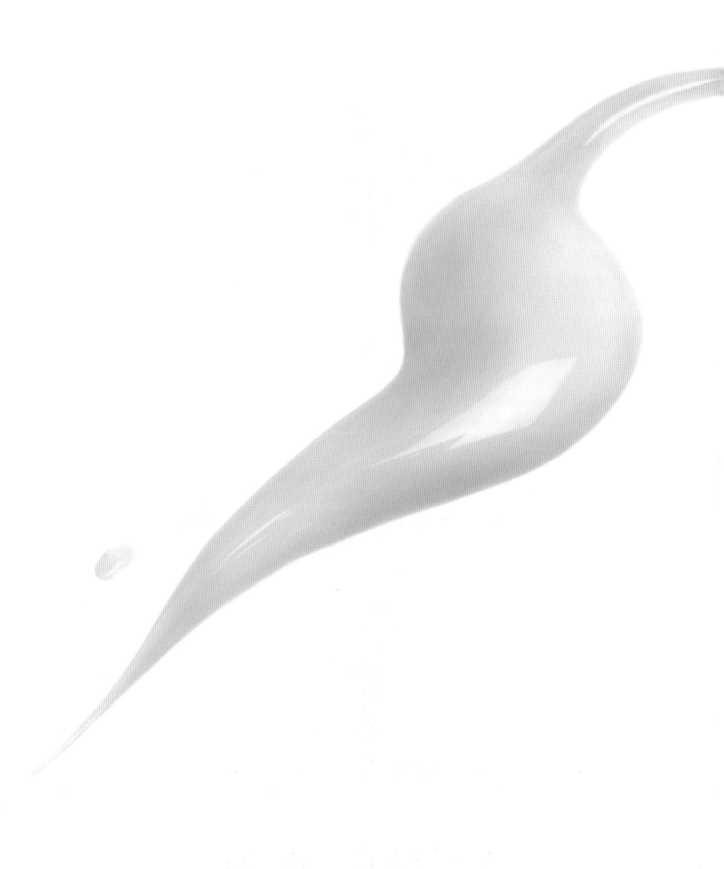

MY BEAUTY CAPITAL

Skin, water: skimming the surface, reflecting my being

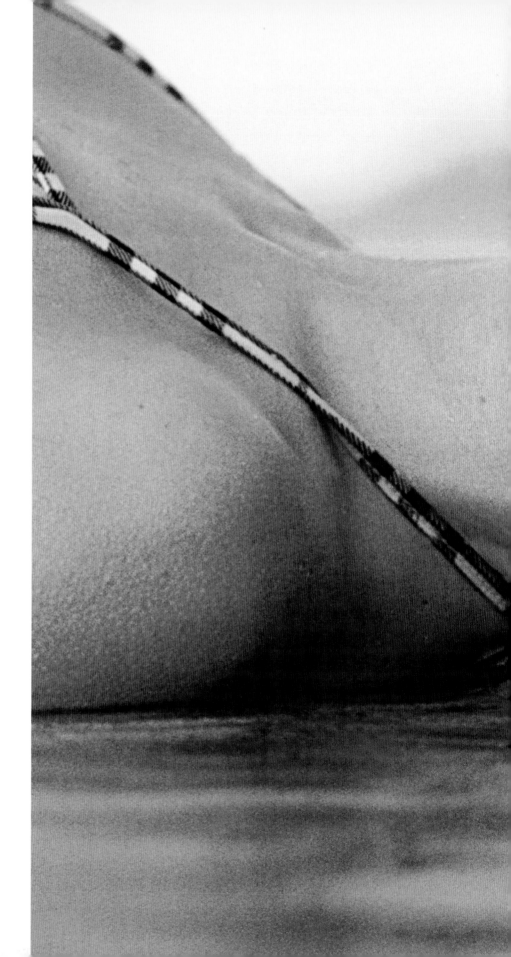

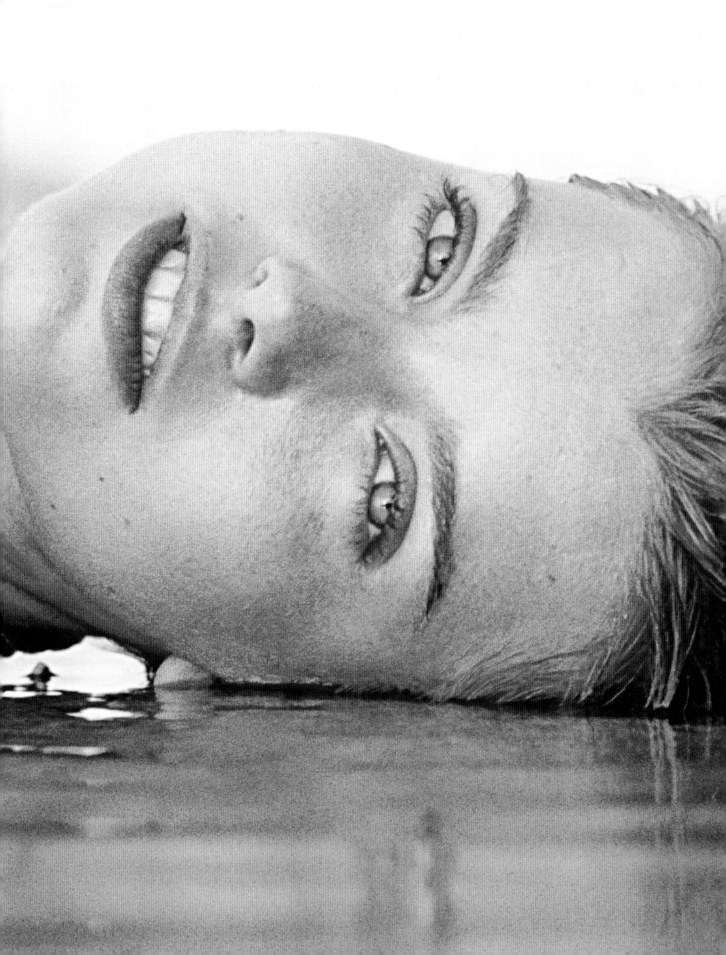

Planet skin its secret life

The body's number-one organ, skin offers the most effective form of security (and survival) blanket. But its incredible resources deserve a guided tour … beneath the surface.

SKIN IS THE MOST INTELLIGENT OF TISSUES

The informative skin …
Cutaneous receptors transmit all the news to the brain in real time: this is soft, that's hot, that stings …

… and the caring skin
Absorbing oxygen and rejecting carbon dioxide, the skin is able to diffuse active ingredients into the bloodstream.
• The proof of collagen's durability? It's what's left of an animal's skin, which we call leather!

THE WORD FROM THE DERMATOLOGIST
The stratum corneum contains on average five to ten 'strata', up to twenty on the back, and up to hundreds on the soles of the feet. The mucous membranes do not have this layer.

At almost 2 m² with a thickness of between 1.5 and 4 mm, and weighing around 3 kilograms, the skin is **our largest vital organ** in volume. A unique combination of 2000 billion hyperactive cells, it protects our entire body.

Skin analyses our whole environment to regulate our body temperature, protect us from cold and heat, block out ultraviolet rays, destroy threatening bacteria and generate antibodies. A vital interface with the external world, it is made up of **three high-protection layers.**

THE EPIDERMIS

With a thickness between 0.05 mm (on the eyelids) to 2–3 mm (on the soles of the feet), the epidermis is in direct contact with the external world. Its mission: to prevent any intruders from penetrating our skin … Its exceptional longevity comes from the perpetual renewal of cells, **keratinocytes**, which are in a permanent state of migration from the **basal cell layer** (the boundary between the epidermis and dermis) toward the surface, where they pile up into little tiles to become **corneocytes.** They take 28 days to 'ripen', developing a protective sheath to make up the **stratum corneum ('horny layer')**, before drying out and flaking off to make room for the new generations.

The **hydrolipidic film**, a mixture of sweat and sebum, ensures the moisture balance of our skin. If this protective covering is threatened, the stratum corneum, which is not as well-hydrated, will thicken and age prematurely. ▶

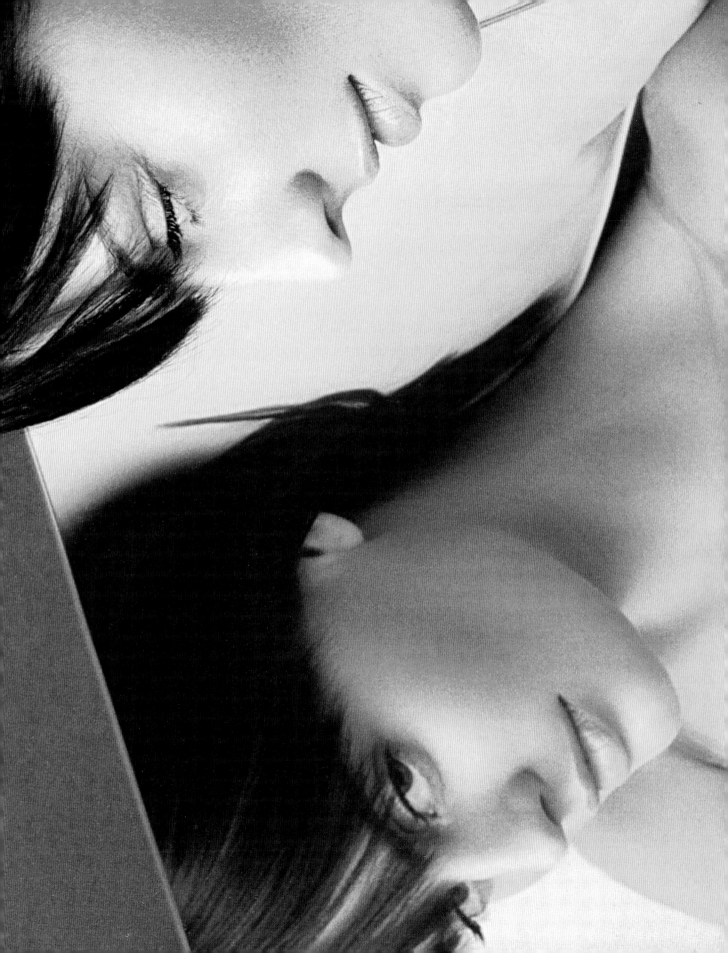

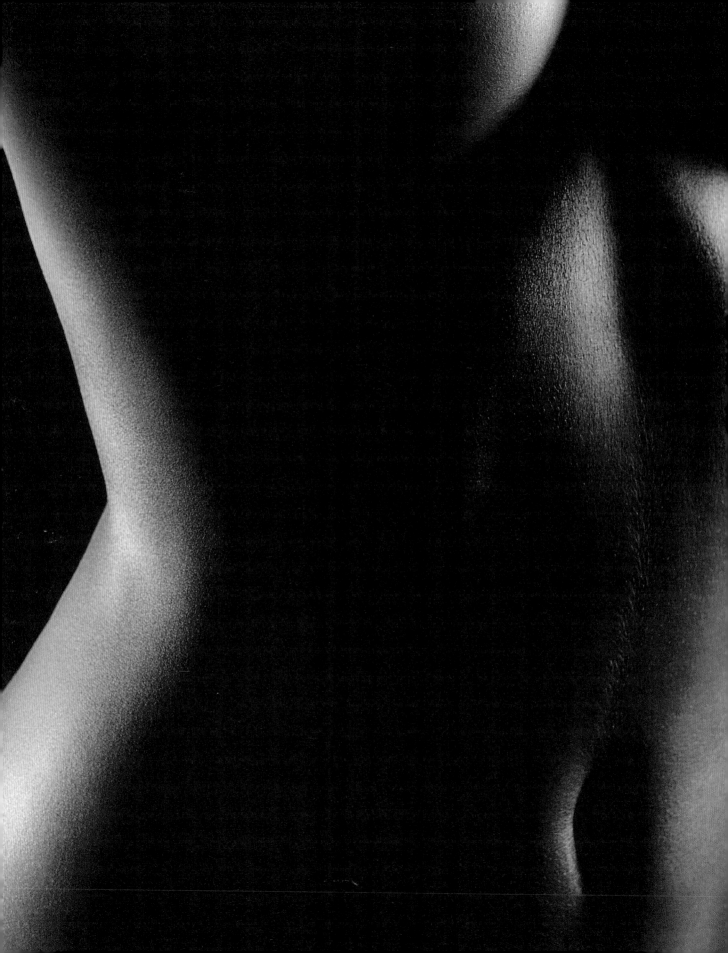

▶ THE DERMIS

This is the skin's thickest layer, both firm and supple: it is the supporting (connective) tissue that underlies the epidermis and gives the skin its consistency, elasticity and tone. Its cells (**fibroblasts**) produce **proteins** that allow for the retention of moisture: **collagen** fibres ensure firmness and **elastin** gives skin its ability to return to its shape after being stretched. But when people talk about the signs of 'cutaneous ageing', they're talking about the dermis! Throughout the dermis are nutrient-bearing blood vessels that feed the epidermis, and countless nerves that faithfully report all the undesirable incidents perceived by the sensors to the brain. They transmit instructions in the event of heat (perspiration), cold (the blood vessels shrink, the skin becomes pale) or shock (ouch!).

THE HYPODERMIS

A shock absorber and 'pantry' for the skin, like a cushion stuffed with **lipids** (fats), located beneath the dermis, the hypodermis has the role of stocking up on reserves which can be available in the event of a lack of food or energy, but it also protects from the cold.

The cells that 'allow' us to store fats, the **adipocytes** (fat cells), are distributed differently according to sex: while they prefer to settle under men's stomachs, they have a predilection for our buttocks and thighs: it's what makes 'gynoid' (womanly) figures what they are—with the (alas) visible result being ... cellulite, the product of this accumulation of fat and water trapped inside the tissues.

Our dermis is made up of 70% water ... The skin contains 25 to 35% of all of our body's water reserves, or 9 litres.

THE WORD FROM THE ANGIOLOGIST
Men have (almost) no cellulite.
Our fatty tissue represents 23% of the weight of the female body, compared to 15% for men. The explanation for this genetic 'injustice'? Women are programmed to ensure the survival of the species!

Express diagnosis
my true nature

*There's no final skin type: your skin evolves, just like you do!
It glows when everything is going well and emits distress signals
in times of stress. It's simply a matter of paying attention to it.*

A 'good' level of hydration of the horny layer of the skin is 13%. If it falls to 10%, the skin is dry.

The lubricating abilities of the sebaceous glands also protect against bacteria; and sebum, together with water, makes up the very precious hydrolipidic film.

THE WORD FROM BÉATRICE BRAUN
Be careful of wearing overly tight clothing, which hinders blood and lymph circulation, leading to the development of cellulite and spider veins, and affects the texture of the skin. The test? When you get undressed, you shouldn't see any marks from your clothes!

NORMAL SKIN

A state of grace (quite rare, take advantage of it!): almost invisible pores, even skin tone, a natural and durable radiance.

COMBINATION SKIN

A shinier **T-zone** (forehead-nose-chin) betrays oilier skin along this key median strip; the skin on the rest of the face may be dry.

OILY SKIN

The only real test: oily traces on a piece of tissue paper applied to clean skin. The symptoms: blackheads (plugs of sebum that is too thick to drain away), while excess stores create pimples. Above all, don't get aggressive with it—instead, show understanding and get medical advice if required.

DRY SKIN

Dry skin is more fragile. The warning sign: if skin feels tight half an hour after cleaning, there's a problem with the hydrolipidic film, and bacteria have free access. On the body, the especially vulnerable zones are elbows, knees and feet.

SENSITIVE SKIN

Irritable and reactive, your skin seems intolerant of everything and uses every shade of the spectrum to tell you about it, as well as tingling sensations. Any level of friction is unbearable. But it can simply be a temporary condition due to pollution or stress. The culprits can be detected with a little patience (it takes two months to be certain whether a product is suitable for the skin) or by deciding to let the skin breathe for a while.

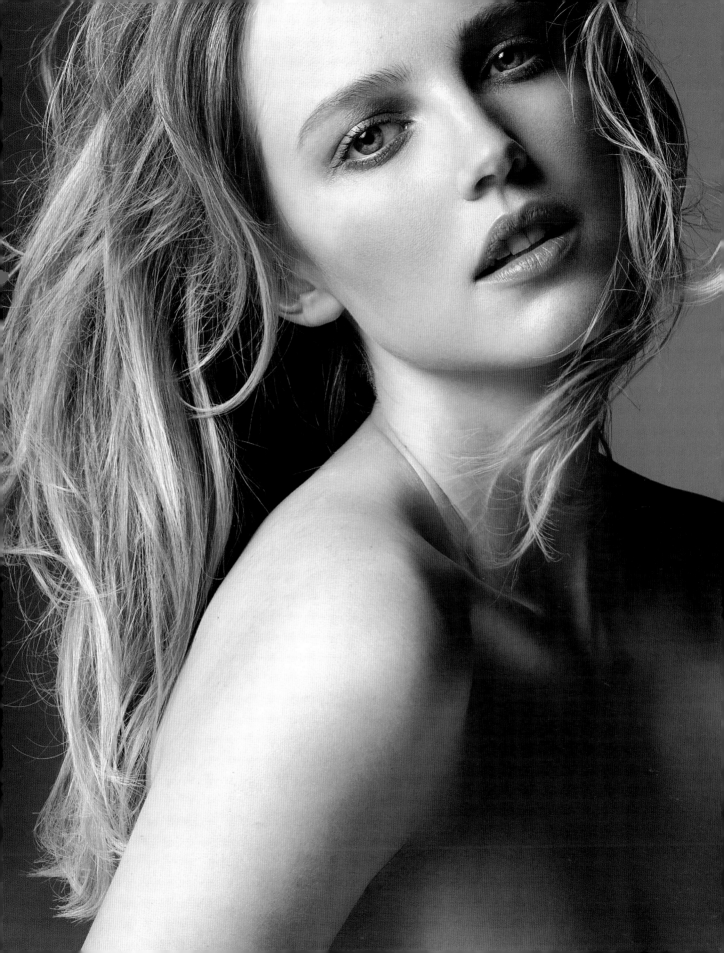

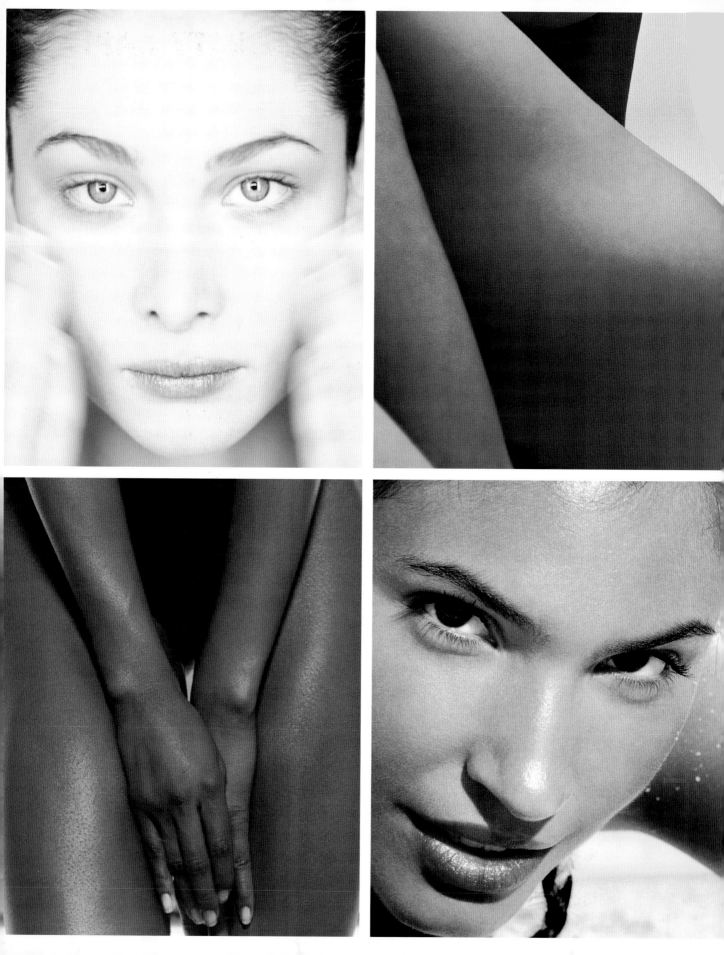

Phototypes
the sun in my skin

We're not all equal under the sun:
melanin divides us according to our reaction to UV rays …

OUR EPIDERMIS IS TRANSPARENT!

The pigment **melanin**, which is produced by our 'tanning' cells, the **melanocytes**, colours our skin to protect us from the sun by creating a **tan** as a sort of natural biological parasol. The dosage of the mixture of **eumelanin** (true black melanin) and **pheomelanin** (orange) explains the fact that every different shade exists under the sun.

SHADES OF SHADE...

Apart from the **4 phototypes**, from very fair to dark, scientists classify us from 1 to 8 (albino, red-haired with milky-white skin, blonde with fair skin, fair-haired with fair skin, chestnut-coloured hair with fair skin, brown hair with dark skin, dark brown hair with dark skin, black), in decreasing order according to the risk faced when exposed to the MED (minimum erythema dose): namely the amount of sun exposure before developing sunburn.

There's an optimum amount for each of us, beyond which the benefits of the sun turn into damage to the skin.

However, not only are our reserves of melanin not inexhaustible (the number of melanocytes **decreases after the age of 30**, so there is less protection from UV rays and the risk of melanoma rises), but their size varies greatly, **by up to 300%**, according to the individual.

And if some parts of the body tan better than others, this is because the skin has a memory. Because the arms are more often exposed to the sun, they are better trained.

The synthesis of vitamin D, which takes place under the effect of ultraviolet rays, is a vital process: it enables calcium to be absorbed by the digestive system and attach to the bones.

The melanocytes, which are responsible for synthesising melanin, have their work cut out for them: there is only one of them per 35 keratinocytes.

THE WORD FROM RESEARCHER GÉRARD REDZINIAK
The epidermis is not powerful enough as a parasol: 30% of 'ageing' UVA rays and 10% of carcinogenic UVB rays manage to reach the dermis!

Beautiful at 20
and at any age

The ideal of eternal beauty—the dream of the modern Cleopatra.
The future of our skin lies deep inside our cells.

MY SKIN'S AGE

There's nothing more alive than the skin … The dream of having the skin of a baby—taut, immaculately fine, with no visible pores (and no sebum)—is over as soon as the hormones wake up and the production of sebum gets under way. The pores open up to allow excess to seborrhoea drain away, and black-heads and pimples can appear in the thickening epidermis.

AT WHAT AGE SHOULD I DECIDE TO PUT TIME INTO REVERSE?

The synthesis of fibres slows down: an ageing skin is one whose fibroblasts—the slatted 'bed-base' of the skin, which support the mattress of the epidermis—are deteriorating. It's the whole apparatus that's best kept in shape, whatever our age! Since our skin 'capital' is laid down between the ages of fifteen and twenty, it's sensible to look ahead: moisturising products are beneficial from adolescence onwards, with an obvious preventative role.

The **mitochondria** are our central power plants, transforming the glucose that results from the digestive process into energy (adenosine triphosphate—ATP) that can be directly used by the cell. They use food to provide 90% of the body's energy, but also produce the **free radicals** responsible for ageing and degenerative diseases: cellular DNA is the object of 10,000 free radical attacks each day! With its accompanying set of irritations—the thickening of the skin's stratum corneum, a reduction in elasticity, the slow-down of cell 'turnover', and a reduction in the activity of the melanocytes—pigment is not as well distributed.

▶

Hormones pass on all the news inside a network that functions like a biological Internet. Information is stored in the hard drive of our cells, the nucleus.

THE HOME TEST
Slack skin? To find out… 10 seconds on the clock! Pinch your cheek or the back of your hand, watch and count. If the fold disappears in under ten seconds, no need to worry. If the mark stays longer, a firming program would be a good idea!

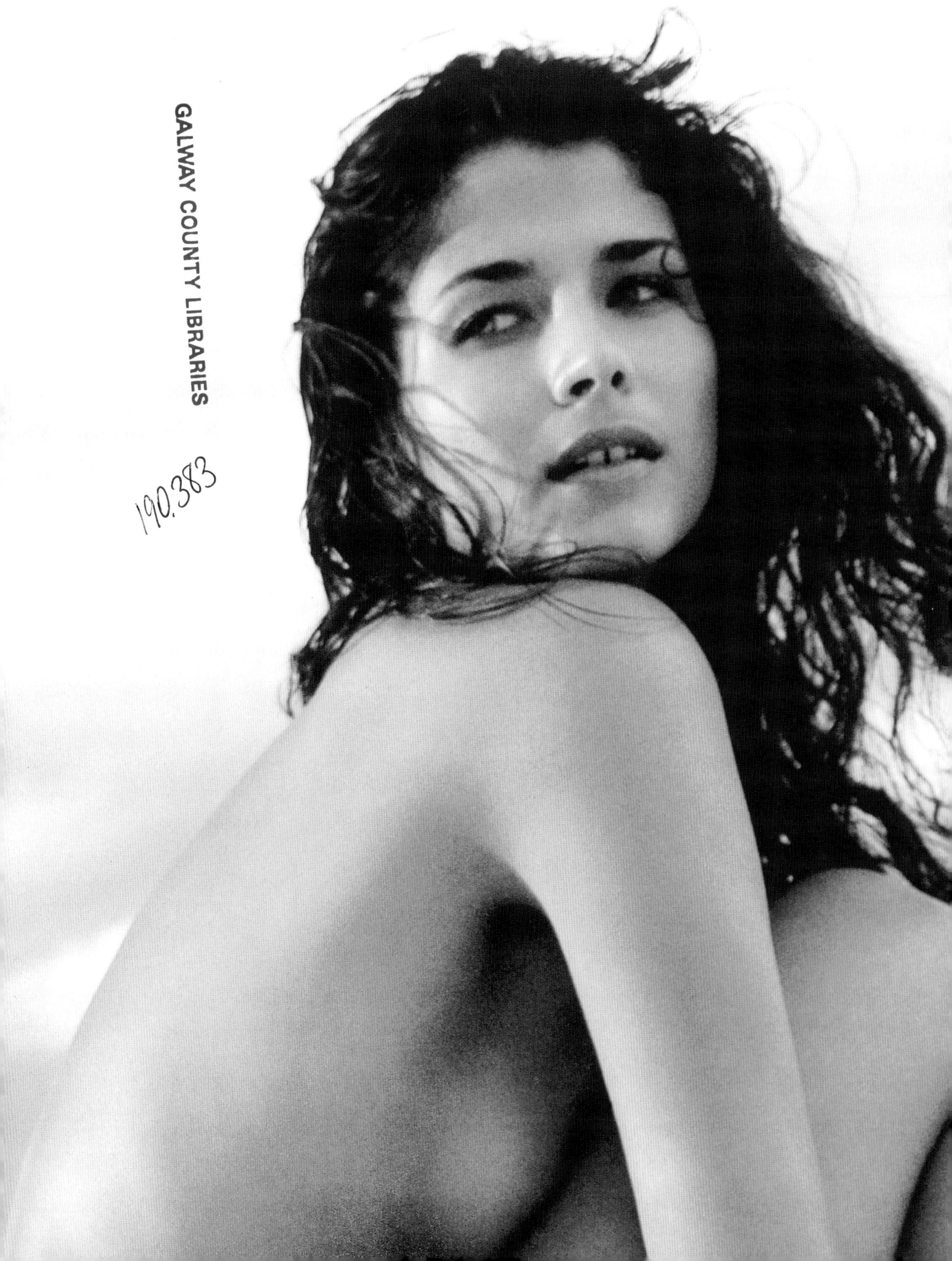

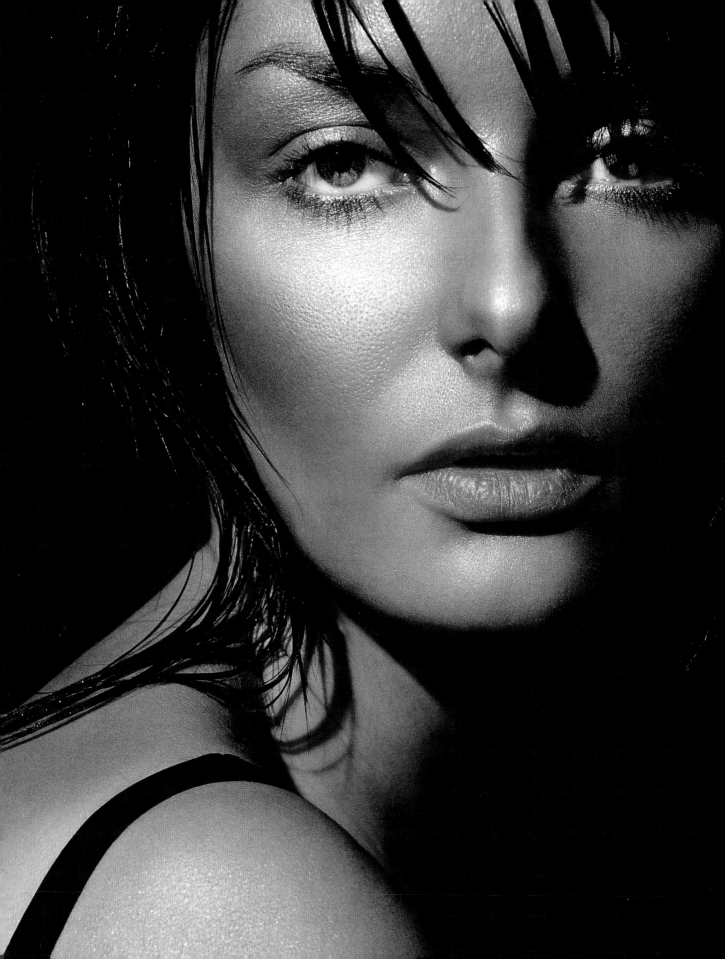

▶ **ADVICE FROM PROFESSOR MARIE-THÉRÈSE LECCIA**

Professor of Dermatology and Photobiology at Grenoble's University Hospital Centre

The **signs of skin ageing**, which we see when we look at ourselves in the mirror (sagging skin or—if you go out into the sun regularly and have dark skin—thickening, yellowing or sunken skin) are, for the overwhelming majority, connected to the sun. Obviously, environment and lifestyle factors must also be taken into account—a balanced diet and as few toxins as possible (alcohol, tobacco … the effects of sunbathing are much worse if you smoke as well!).

The key issue in all of these 'rearrangements' (structural changes) is **oxidative stress**, the overproduction of reactive types of oxygen.

These 'reactive molecules' derived from oxygen are constantly produced within our cells and are normally eliminated. But when there are certain environmental changes (exposure to ultraviolet radiation, temperature, toxins and pollutants …), their production gets out of control and they become aggressive.

They then attack not only the cell itself (DNA, membranes, proteins) but also its environment, the whole of the tissue structure. Thus, at the level of the dermis they degrade the molecules that give skin its lovely texture, in particular collagen and elastin fibres.

This overproduction creates an imbalance in relation to the defence mechanisms (the antioxidant defences one normally has to protect the skin)—and it is this imbalance, as it gets worse, that causes the skin to age.

Hormonal treatments for menopause will correct the hormonal changes that can be expressed on the level of the skin (loss of tone, sagging), but also changes in one's energy and wellbeing, which can lead to slight depression, sleep disturbances or other disorders.
Treatments are adapted to the specific case and administered under strict medical supervision.

The future
in skin

According to Professor Laurent Misery, director of the skin neurobiology laboratory in Brest, France, and a specialist in the links between the skin and the brain, the power of neurotransmitters opens up exciting new paths for the future of cosmetology ...

THE PROMISE OF NEURO-COSMETICS

All of the skin's functions are controlled by the nervous system and thus the mind: **neurotransmitters** (chemical messengers) relay information between the skin and the nervous system, which mostly plays a balancing role, except in the case of certain dermatological diseases or cosmetic inflammatory problems, when it can aggravate the condition, triggering skin problems (reactive skin).

Cosmetic preparations based on 'neuro-psycho-dermatology', by acting on a neurotransmitter (whether by reinforcing or countering its action), could have a great deal to contribute:

• **anti-inflammatory**, soothing sensitive skins, suppressing itching and tingling.

• **anti-hair loss**, halting the process of hair loss.

• **anti-cellulite**, the development of fat cells being very much connected to neurotransmitters such as **VIP** (vasoactive intestinal peptide) and **leptin**, a protein released by adult fat cells that informs the brain about fatty tissue reserves (a product arising from research on neuropeptides is in fact already on the market).

• **anti-age spots**, by envisaging the repigmentation of depigmented zones (and vice versa). On the other hand, it doesn't yet seem possible to reprogram the whole skin surface in order, for example, to give yourself an entirely new phototype.

• **anti-age**, by stimulating the neurotransmitters that encourage the **synthesis of collagen and elastin**.

Long live the neuro-psycho-sensory!
The actual practice of taking care of oneself, of using cosmetics, results in pleasurable sensations, already contributing a little to wellbeing. Thus, the action of massage by itself is enough to increase natural levels of **dopamine**, which transmits pleasure on the cerebral level.

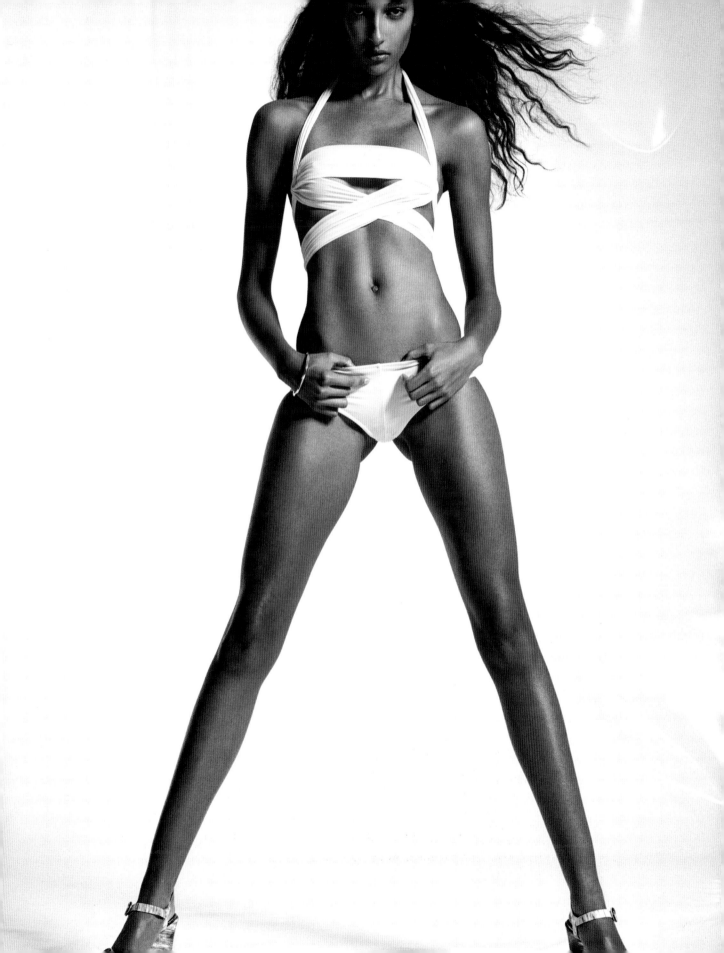

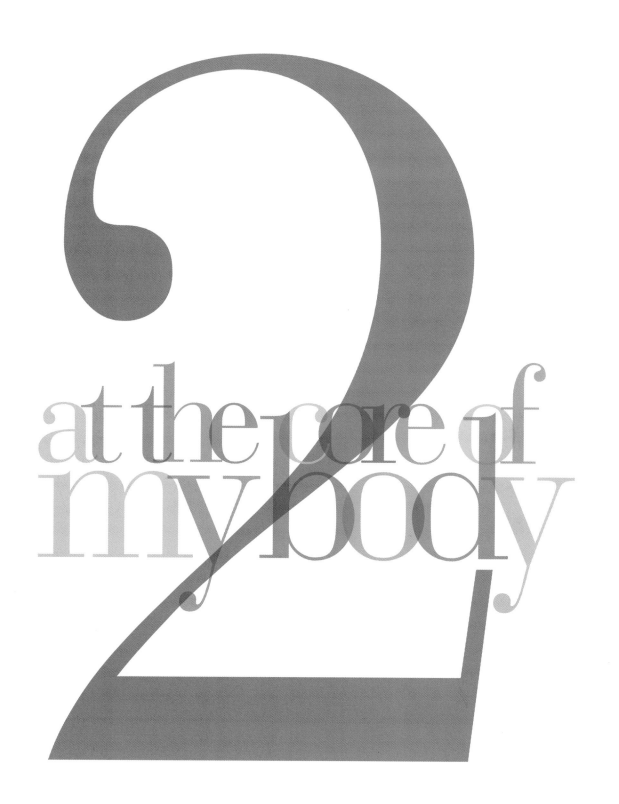

2

at the core of my body

THE DETAILS IN CLOSE-UP

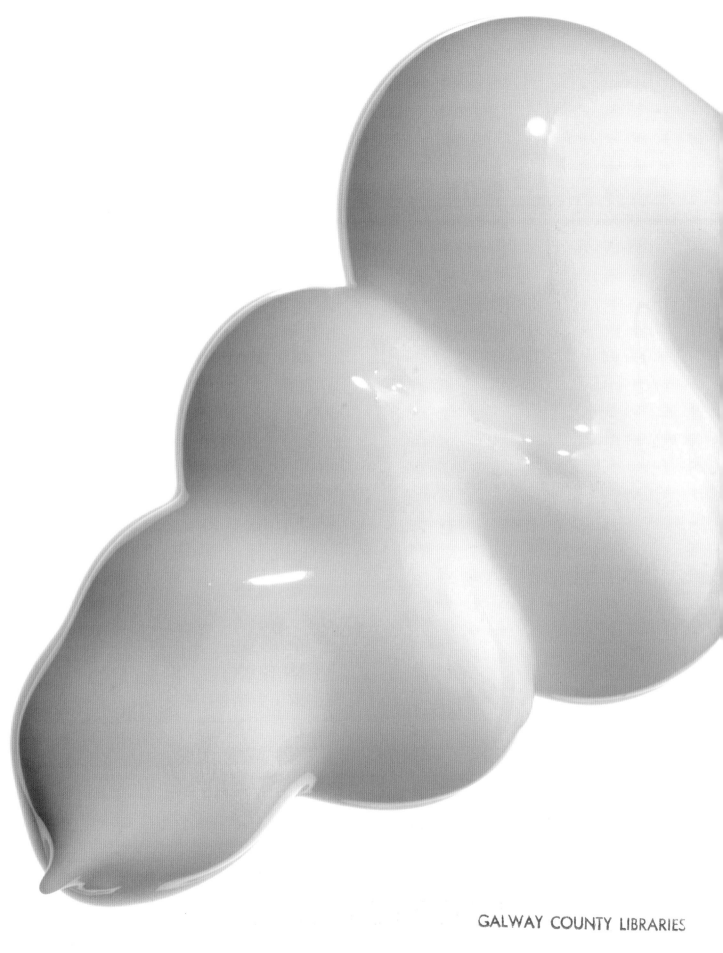

THE DETAILS IN CLOSE-UP

Exploring my palette to discover my best features

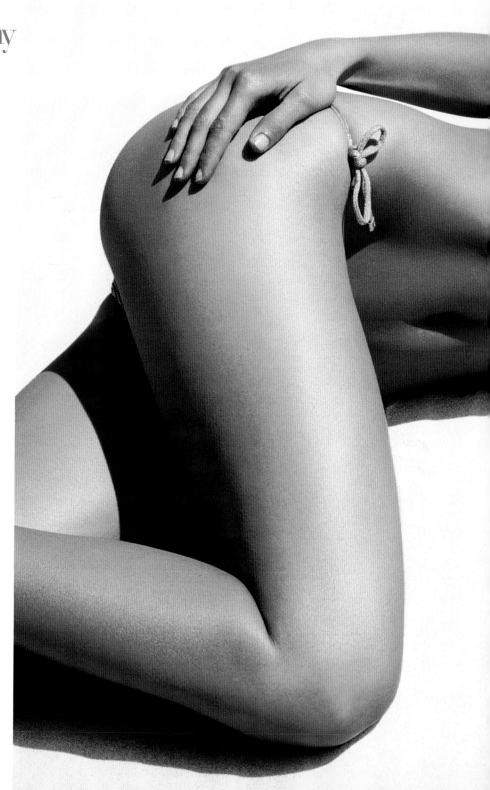

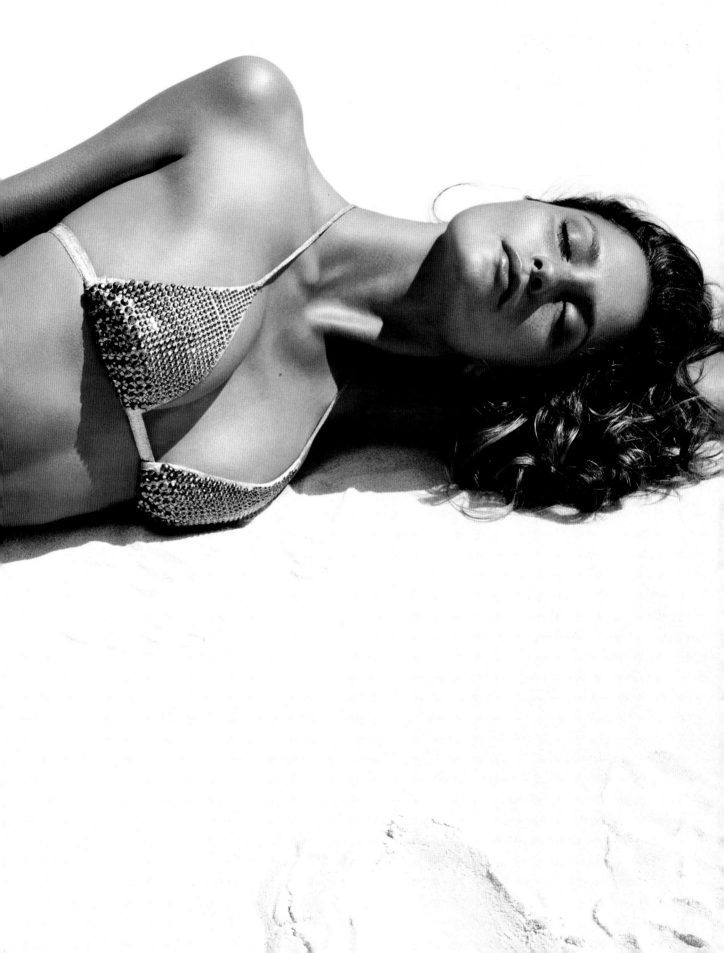

Perfect poise…
elegant neck

Slender or strong, the line of the neck gives you the bearing of a queen. It is also extremely vulnerable and betrays the signs of age that a smooth face is quite capable of hiding!

Bare nape and neck for attracting kisses
Ideal spots for a drop of perfume.

THE WORD FROM THE COACH
• Sitting on a chair with the back nice and straight, draw 10 ovals with the point of the nose by moving the head from front to back, then rest for 10 seconds with the head tilted back. Do the same thing to the right and to the left, vertically and horizontally.
• Support the back of the neck when watching television
• Light summer and winter scarves
• Hot showers for getting out kinks in the neck
TO BE AVOIDED BY ALL NECKS!
• very large pillows
• draughts

AHEAD BY A NECK

Supple and graceful, with incredible mobility, the neck nevertheless bears the heavy burden of keeping your chin up … by supporting no fewer than 5 kg (the weight of the brain). A challenge that is all the greater given that **its musculature is not as dense as that of the face, and its skin is as fine as the skin around the eyes** and very low in sebum. It must not be neglected in one's **daily moisturing and nourishing regime**, because even if it doesn't wrinkle, it can lose its elasticity and take on a 'wobbly' appearance. So, morning and evening, indulge in extra-nourishing preparations enriched with astringent properties, which tighten and support the skin by creating protective films that have a lifting effect.

SOS double chin Preparations with slimming and draining ingredients help to restore facial definition, while lifting and firming preparations strengthen the support tissue.

Anti-sagging The micro-infiltration of placental extracts can revitalise and thus improve the consistency of the skin's structure.

REGAL BEARING

Walk straight ahead with your elbows in your palms, behind the back, shoulder blades squeezed together: nothing better for realigning the spinal column. Also: face gym (page 157).

TURN HEADS

Long neck—a mid-length haircut and as much neck decoration as you like. **Short neck**—keep the nape bare and no turtlenecks.

Thick neck—hair up, plunging necklines, drop earrings.

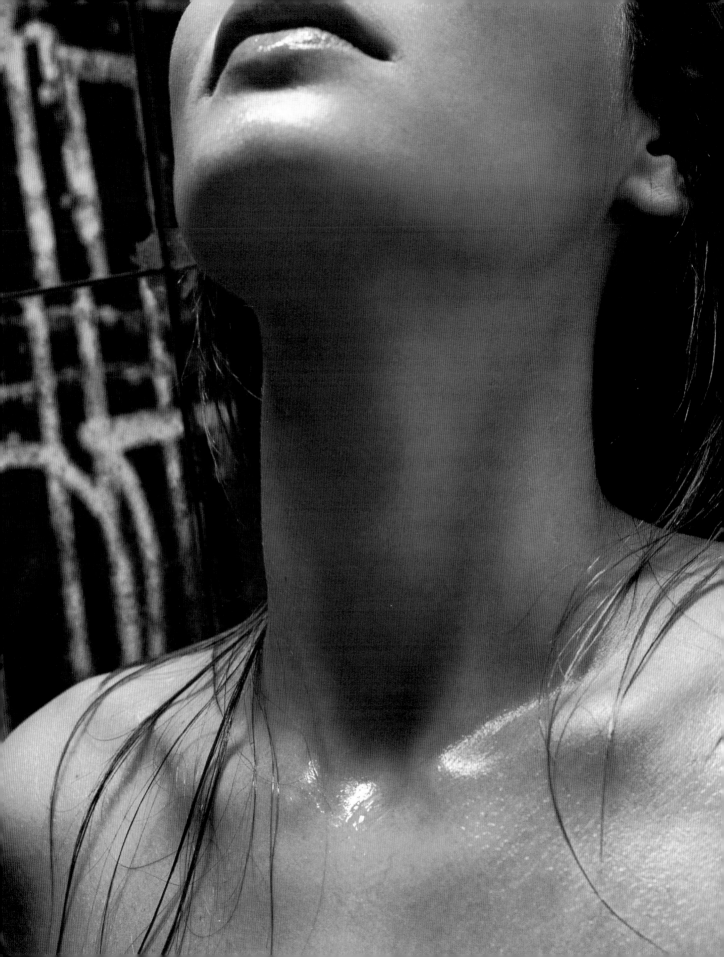

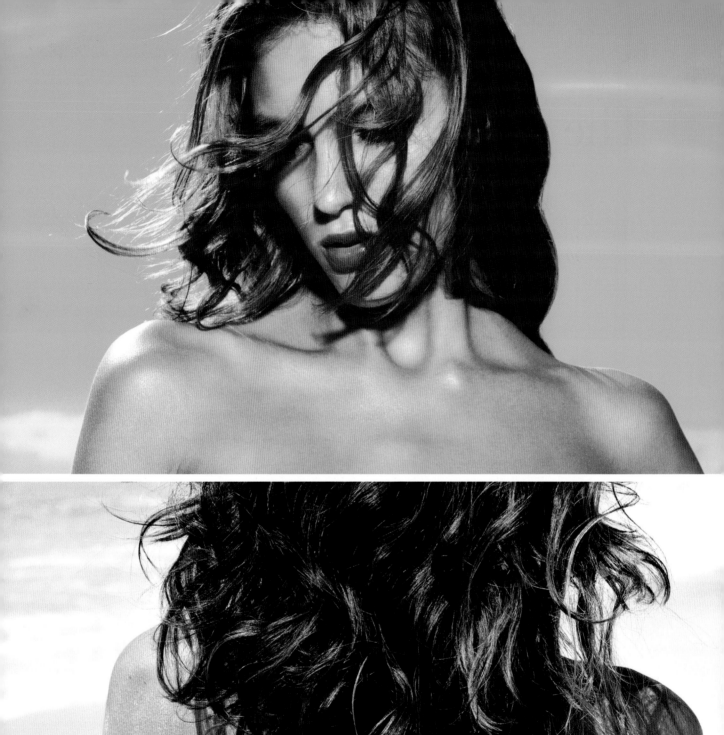
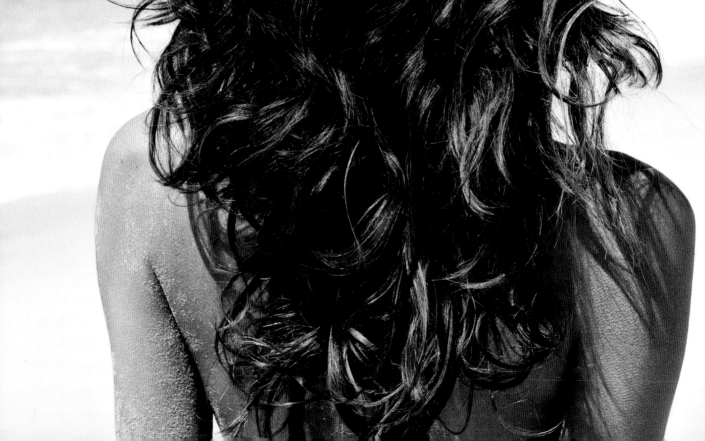

The low-down
on shoulders

They give form to the figure, supporting the whole architecture of the body, defining our stance and summing up our whole outlook on life. A single motto: shoulders back … everyone!

SQUARE, SCULPTURAL SHOULDERS ARE IN VOGUE

It's a very good idea to keep one's head on one's shoulders. It's hard to imagine a more ingenious arrangement than this incredibly complex joint, connecting the shoulder blade (scapula) to the upper arm (humerus), and kept supple by an interplay of ligaments.

Lovely shoulders, solid and well developed, set off the figure and help us to stand nice and straight.

Good posture — with shoulders loose and held well back — opens up the chest and makes breathing easier. Stand up nice and straight, stretch and smoothly roll the shoulders.

There are lots of good exercises for shoulder tone and flexibility. When it comes to sport, it all depends on what kind of figure you have.

If you have shoulders that are too narrow, swimming is the supreme sport for creating lovely shoulders, as is tennis.

If you have shoulders that are too wide, give yourself dancer's legs or take up sports that involve sliding or gliding, from skiing to rollerskating.

STAND-OUT SHOULDERS

Square Tank-tops, strapless tops, halter tops, boat-neck tops will show off well-defined shoulders.

Sloping Besides shoulder pads, you can cheat to give yourself breadth across the shoulders by adding fullness.

Computer mouses: Manipulate while keeping elbows flat on the desk. Without any support, it's the equivalent of weighing 5 kg of stress on the muscles and, in the long term, damaging the cervical vertebrae.

THE WORD FROM THE COACH

PERSONAL MASSAGES
• Starting from the neck, knead the upper edge of the shoulders between the palm and fingers, giving special attention to any painful parts, until you reach the arms.
• Massage the shoulder-blades with your fingertips, using small circles.

TENDONITIS
One of the most common forms of shoulder pain is due to the inflammation of the tendons which surround the joint.

Décolletage taking the plunge

Suggestive or just a suggestion, plunging or pushed up, the décolletage is a fashion focal point that's increasingly coming into its own, unabashed, in all seasons ...

Neglecting one's décolletage is out of the question: it needs as much pampering and hydration as the face.

Massage the area by making circles with your fingertips, from the base of the breasts up to the chin, to improve circulation and tone the tissue.

Full throttle! Freshen the décolletage with an exfoliation treatment. Products based on fruit acids will work wonders.

WARNING: FRAGILE

This zone is very sensitive to UV rays: it's often a favourite target for cases of sunburn. And, without (high) protection, too much exposure over the long term results in both elastin and collagen damage, which ends up becoming visible as vertical grooves from collarbone to breast.

WEIGHT TO GO!

There's no question, of course, of muscling up the breasts themselves ... But you can still strengthen the minor and major pectoral muscles that support the chest and open up the ribcage to show the chest to its best advantage.

View... with balcony
• To show off a pretty summer décolletage: oils and glitter.
• To give the impression of volume: a touch of bronzing powder in the hollow between the breasts.
• Special effects: invisible silicone pads, discreetly slipped into the bra.
• To distract attention from very small breasts, use V-necks and collars.

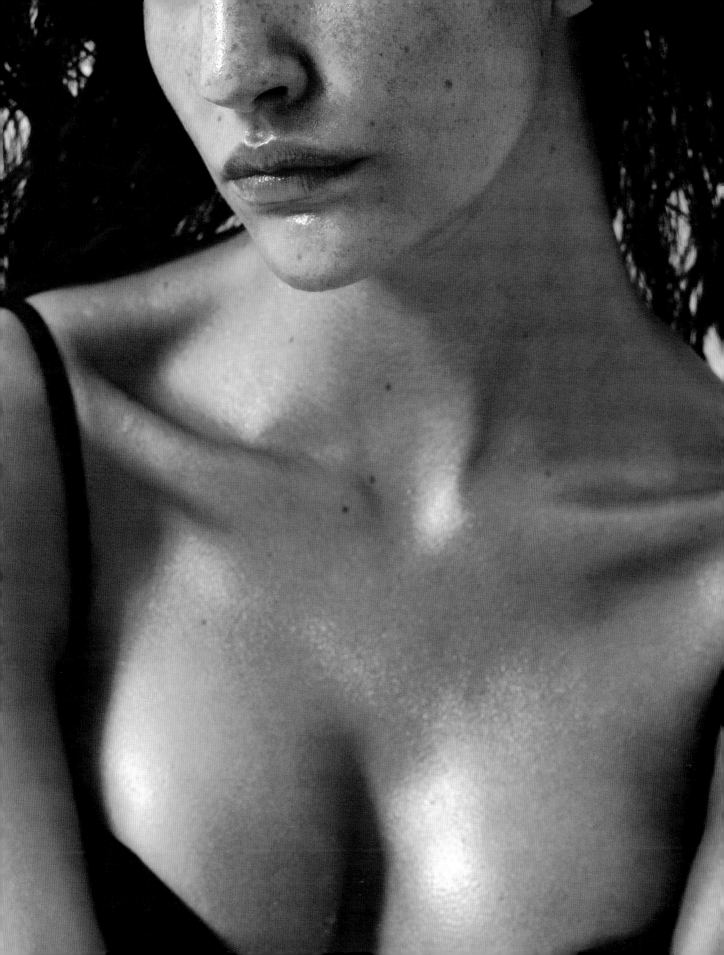

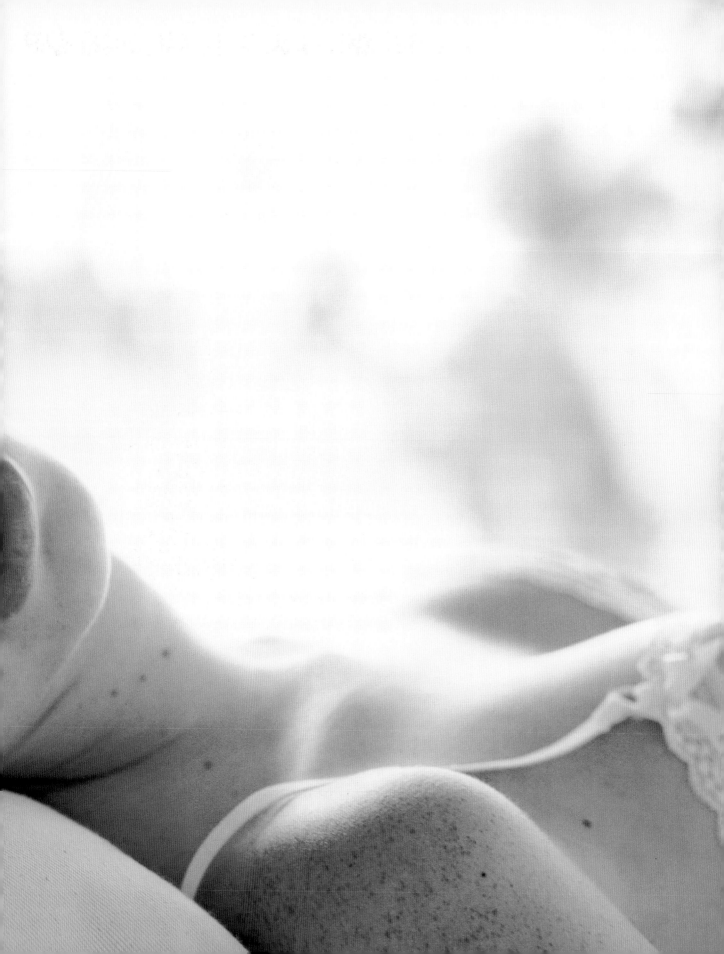

My breasts: the peaks of seduction

Apple or pear shaped, forbidden fruit or bold symbols of femininity, from the smallest to the most generous, their personality has never before been so proudly on display!

THE SKIN, A NATURAL BRASSIERE

Breasts do not contain any muscle and just 'sit' on the chest: only the envelope of the skin, wrapped around the mammary glands, helps them to foil gravity. So stay vigilant!

A COLD SHOWER EVERY DAY: THE BREAST MEDICINE!

A **shower regime** is a must: splash your breasts every day, starting with tepid water, then cool, then cold, massaging gently … it activates the circulation and stimulates the tissues. Excess heat is their greatest enemy!

Always moisturise and tone this fragile area using **circular massaging movements**. Firming treatments and booster masks will stimulate the production of collagen and elastin.

THE RIGHT POSITION

No more rounded backs: sit with your back up straight and your shoulders locked back—it's the best way to avoid the dreaded sag.

SUPPORT COMMITTEE

For everyday A full-cup bra will hold in place even ample chests and offer protection against vibrations from walking.

For sport Crop-top style, reinforced, with wide straps.

For charm Push-up bras artfully shape and lift.

THE KEY POINTS The **back strap** mustn't ride up, the **cups** must be adjusted down to the millimetre, without squashing so they don't hamper circulation. Yes to underwire, as long as it doesn't pinch or hurt. The **shoulder straps**, flat against the hollow of the shoulders, mustn't leave any marks or redness on the skin.

The golden triangle
18 cm from one nipple to another and 18 cm from the nipple to the dip of the collarbone.

THE WORD FROM THE COACH
Sports that build the back and pectoral muscles (swimming, handball …) or targeted exercises:
• lying on your back, holding a 1 kg weight in each hand, knees bent up on the stomach, without arching, slowly lower your arms straight behind your head, then raise just as slowly (20 times).
• lying flat on your stomach, the arms slightly away from the body, palms down and feet pointed, lift the whole body parallel to the ground.
• on your knees, arms stretched out in front, hands on the ground, lower the chin to the ground and raise it slowly.

Harmony is back

Be just as seductive from the back, where we often store tiredness and stress. Toned, relaxed, taken in hand, our back asks only to be forgotten about ...

THE SPINAL COLUMN, A GIFTED GUIDE

Its **joints** adapt to the whole range of bends, stretches and turns, and all kinds of breathing rhythms. The whole apparatus is maintained by ligaments and bundles of muscles which envelop this mechanical—and aesthetic—wonder.

Seduce from behind by keeping your back silky and toned, a sign of strength.

THE SKIN ON THE BACK

Even if it is thicker than the skin on the face, it's still thirsty for cleansing and moisturising. But scrubbing, massaging and moisturising the back are not at all a straightforward matter, even if you're very flexible. A long-handled and soft-bristled brush or horsehair exfoliating strap will help you to exfoliate and massage your back with ease under the shower.

At the beautician's

Purifying and exfoliating treatments, to take care of any pimples and blackheads (steam treatments) and masks (clay, mud, seaweed) for deep cleansing, before moisturising. A massage will provide the finishing touch by stimulating the circulation.

BACK BEAUTIFUL

Backstroke swimming (which builds muscle lengthways), **horse riding** (for posture), **volleyball** and **basketball** (for the stretch that gives uplift to the silhouette). **Yoga** and **pilates** develop the muscles harmoniously while improving flexibility and releasing tensions.

THE WORD FROM THE EXPERT

• Sleep on your back or side, the neck well supported with a small pillow, the spinal column aligned.
• At the office: adjust your seat so that your eyeline is at the height of the screen and stretch regularly, shoulders back.
• In the car: support the back well, the knees level and aligned with the hips, both hands on the steering wheel, arms parallel.

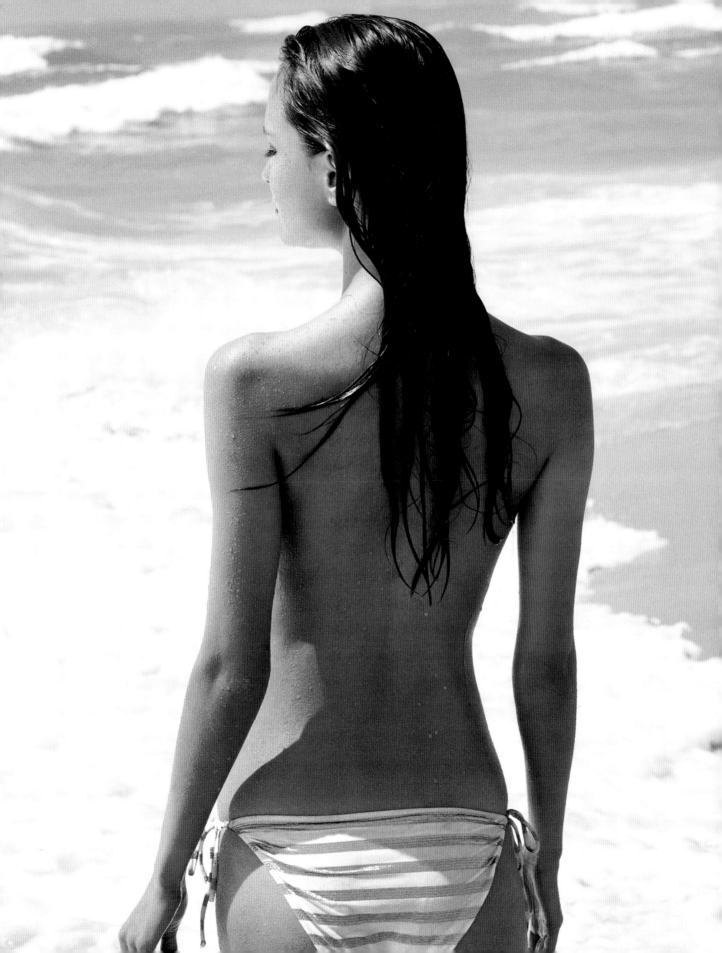

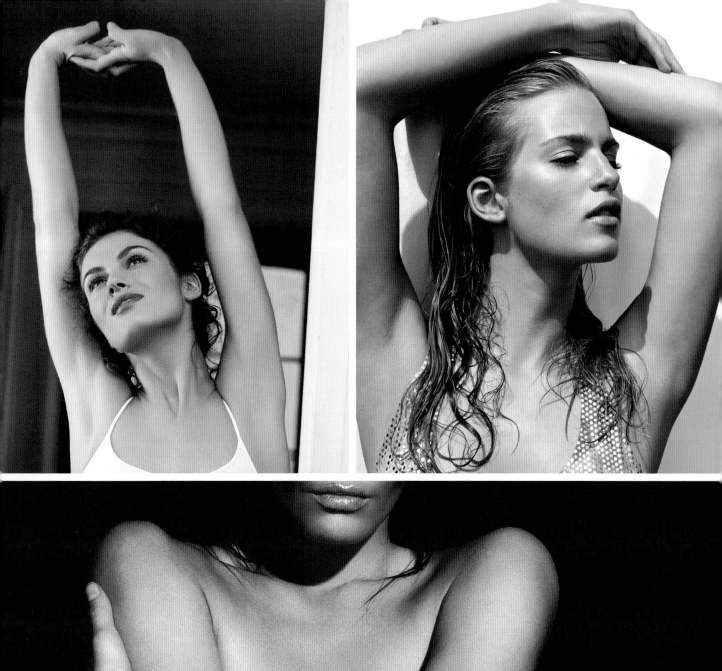
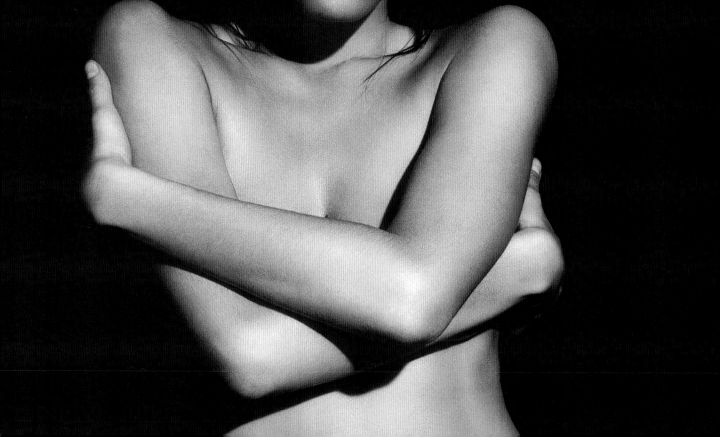

A call to arms

No question of laying down your arms, or sitting on your hands: beautiful arms hold your figure ... at arm's length!

BEAUTIFUL, FEMININE ARMS

They may be bared on any occasion, so all the more reason to keep a firm grip on their appearance! Our body movements are an essential part of the image we project.

The **ultra-fine skin**, especially on the back of the arms, requires special attention with treatments that nourish, firm (it's the first area to show signs of sag), tone and protect. The backs of the arms are **exfoliated** with a crepe glove (horsehair is too harsh), then massaged liberally after showering, moving up from the wrist to the elbow, then from the elbow to the shoulder. **Cellulite** can be curbed in this area as well, using **pinch-and-roll** and **circular massage** techniques with slimming creams.

The elbows really lap up moisturing and nourishing creams—don't let them become chapped and rough.

Downy hair is charming, especially its golden version in summer: unless it is really excessive, bleaching is without question preferable to hair removal.

ARMFULS OF EXERCISE!

Arms turn out to be significantly more responsive than thighs when they're called on. Want muscled arms in a month? Customised exercises firm up the support tissue and resculpt a limp upper arm. Its fat melts away much more quickly than on the legs (instructions at right, to be performed with a pair of adjustable weights).

Dancing to sculpt the figure and develop gracefulness in your movements. **Tennis** and **swimming**; **yoga** once again.

THE WORD FROM THE COACH
SLIMMING REGIME
3 kg in each hand (more than that and you're pumping iron)
• on a chair, knees bent, legs slightly apart, arms loose alongside the body, raise your arms slowly, straight, to shoulder level, then lower slowly (2x20).
IRON ARMS
1.5 kg in each hand for triceps of steel:
• back supported by a chair, raise the left arm, straight up beside the ear
• bend the elbow, bringing the forearm down behind the neck, then raise, straightening the arm
• repeat on the right-hand side (3x30).

My hands
at my fingertips!

They communicate as much through the way they move as in their beauty. The most extraordinary instrument that nature has placed at our disposal ... deserving our full attention.

Hands up!

A study published by the American Society of Plastic Surgeons (ASPS) in June 2006 shows that the best way to guess somebody's age is to look at their... hands! Good news: using nail varnish and wearing jewellery makes them look younger.

The nails

grow 4 mm per month (they are completely renewed in 4 to 6 months), more quickly in warmer weather and on the right hand for right-handed people.

THE WORD FROM THE DERMATOLOGIST

Washing your hands before and after meals (and always after using the toilet), is a public health necessity. And why not protect them with gloves and a layer of cream, even when you're just doing the dishes.

MAINTENANCE IS A MUST!

A perfect and complex mechanism, comprising the supple wrist joint, the five metacarpal (hand) bones, the fingers (two phalanx bones for the thumb, three for the rest) and the many small muscles that give the hand strength and precision: the abductor muscles allowing us to spread the fingers, the adductor muscles to bring them together.

The hands have **thick skin on the palm**, with no sebaceous glands, but **fine skin on the back** and a need for attention that is all the greater because washing the hands dries them out. Gentle, frequent exfoliating scrubs, and daily massage using **special hand creams** for moisturising, nourishing, eliminating age spots. Anti-UV protection is a must.

Special beauty sleep Try an 'intensive' mask treatment, applied in a generous layer and covered with a cotton glove.

For the nails The nails and their lunulae (the 'half-moons') require constant care and vigilance. A strengthening base, and varnish for protection.

SOS breaking nails Ten minutes in a bath of lukewarm sweet almond oil.

Cold snap To facilitate the circulation of the blood back towards the heart, hold the hands in the air and massage, starting from the fingertips and moving up to the wrist.

YOUTH WITHIN HANDS' REACH

Laser treatments and chemical peels can erase brown spots; injections promise to give back the plump look of a baby's hands ...

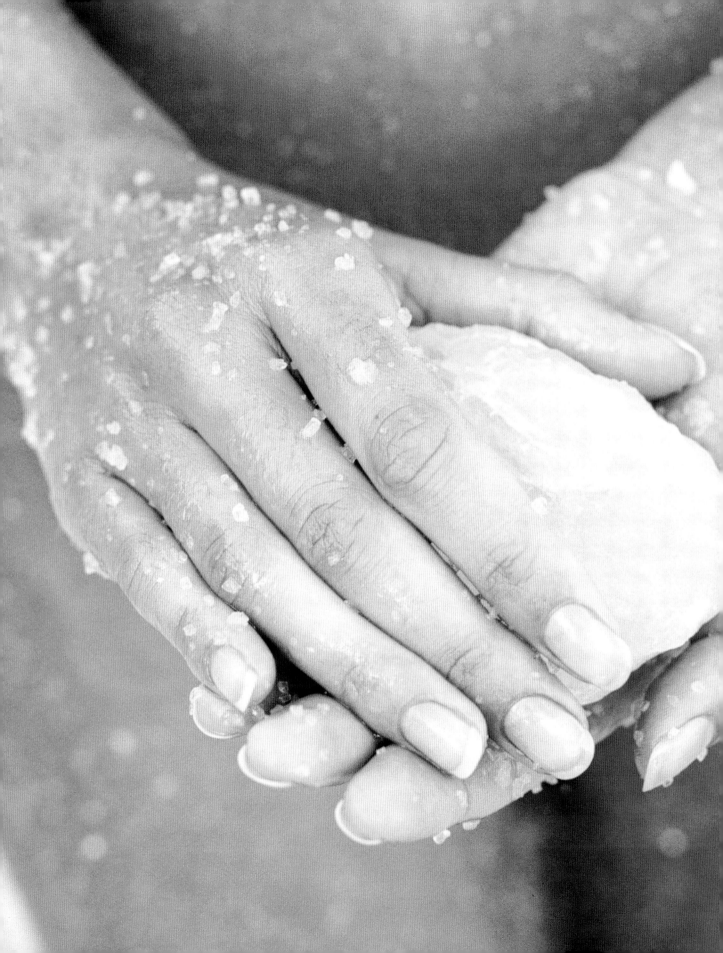

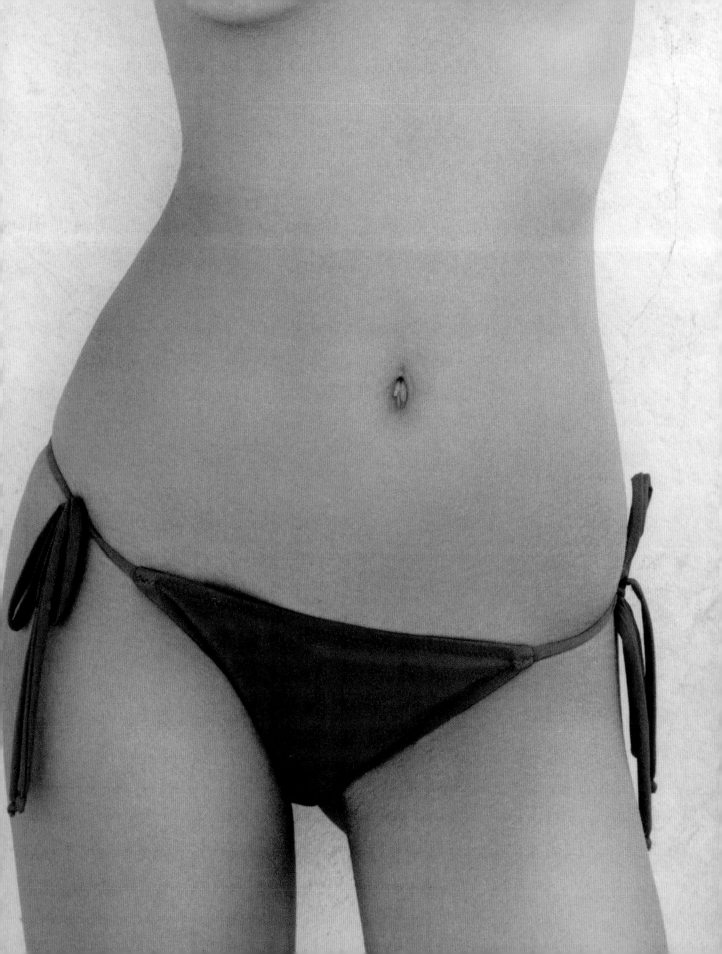

The stomach: waist management

Whether a flat stomach or cute little potbelly, it leads the dance of seduction—especially when low-rise fashions bare it for all to admire …

WASP WAIST Our waist slims down at puberty and thickens at menopause: located 3 cm above the navel, this magic latitude corsets the figure. A pronounced waist has always been a symbol of femininity, but how fine it is also depends on heredity. You can be predisposed to gain weight around the stomach… or the thighs!

NO SLACK FOR THE ABDOMINALS

A swelling tummy ain't always swell … And yet, the female anatomy is predisposed to it: it's a magnet for fat cells. Supporting our efforts in the quest for a flat stomach are two sets of four muscles (the rectus abdominis, external and internal oblique, transverse) which support the abdominal wall and serve as vital protectors of our organs, while at the same time supporting the lower back and helping the spinal column do its job.

Apart from green tea-based detox programs combined with an appropriate diet, daily exercise is the only way to give yourself abs of reinforced steel, by limiting the fatty tissue and boosting the supporting muscular girdle—even after having a baby, once the perinaeum has returned to normal.

Targeted ab exercises (with variations, so you don't get bored) and massages using **fluid-draining formulas** (caffeine, bitter orange, calcium) which lift the skin and sculpt the abdomen.

Pinch-and-roll! At home or at the beautician's, stomach cellulite is controlled by repeated massaging, whereby it's squeezed and rolled between the hands, alternated with effleurage and concentric massage movements in a clockwise direction.

The golden figure: 0.7 the ideal chest-waist-hips ratio (for example 90-63-90)

Eat slowly
Exercise
Breathe deeply
The trifecta for toning the stomach.

THE WORD FROM THE COACH
KEEP THE STOMACH IN WHEN YOU GO OUT
When walking, remember to pull in the navel, lower the ribs and squeeze the buttocks!

THE KING OF AB EXERCISES
• lying on your back, legs straight up in the air, breathe in deeply then lift the upper body while breathing out slowly and looking at the ceiling to raise the back without curling the neck. At the end of the exhalation 'pull' the navel toward the spinal column.

FLAT STOMACH RECIPES
• Rowing, canoeing and backstroke strengthen the abdominal belt.
• Pilates, queen of stomach exercises, and yoga.
• Best of the (flat) belly dances, the salsa!

Femininity in the saddle

The small of the back is big news!
Sitting down on the job is out of the question: beautiful buttocks change the face of the world!

BOOTY BOMBSHELL: A SOLID CHOICE

The preferred shape is full, high and rounded, African-style, which means not letting up the pressure! The good news: it's the **quality of the skin, a true natural girdle**, that gives the butt its cheeky profile. So the most important thing in this area is to stimulate the circulation and tone of the skin … which is much easier than changing one's body type.

THE BOTTOM LINE

Gluteus maximus, medius and minimus A trio of muscles for shaping a dreamy set of curves: the gluteus minimus and medius (abductor muscles) take care of the sides, outlining the hips, the gluteus maximus, the rounded part. To know where you sit, here are three types …

Generous bottom (endomorph) A spectacular rear, but soon vulnerable to the threat of gravity if the gluteus maximus acquires a layer of fat, a victim of the 'just one (chocolate) won't make a difference' syndrome.

Flat buttocks (mesomorph) firm and well-defined, but not very rounded.

Under-developed buttocks (ectomorph): curves can be sought from targeted exercises.

THE SPECIAL TOUCH

Pinch-and-roll massages accompanied by smoothing and draining treatments of all kinds are just the thing. Daily massages, always in an upward direction, to lift and boost the whole area.

THE WORD FROM THE COACH
MODEL EXERCISES
• Think about squeezing your buttocks together at all times, training yourself to tense them for longer and longer periods.
• Walk with long steps, pushing off the back leg.
• Boycott escalators and elevators. EVERYTHING GETS A LIFT
• Lying on your right side, right leg bent, upper body leaning towards the ground, the left leg stretched, with the foot pointing downwards. Breathe in deeply, then breathe out, pushing the left leg back without arching the back (x 25 each leg).
• Lying on your back, raise the legs slowly to the vertical, toes pointed (x 25).

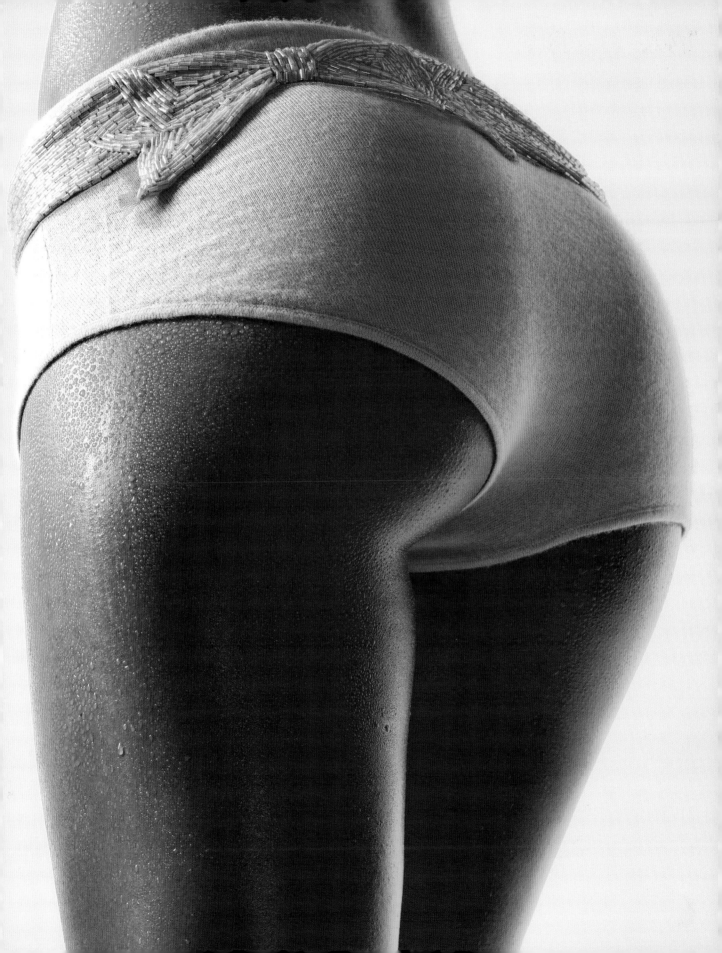

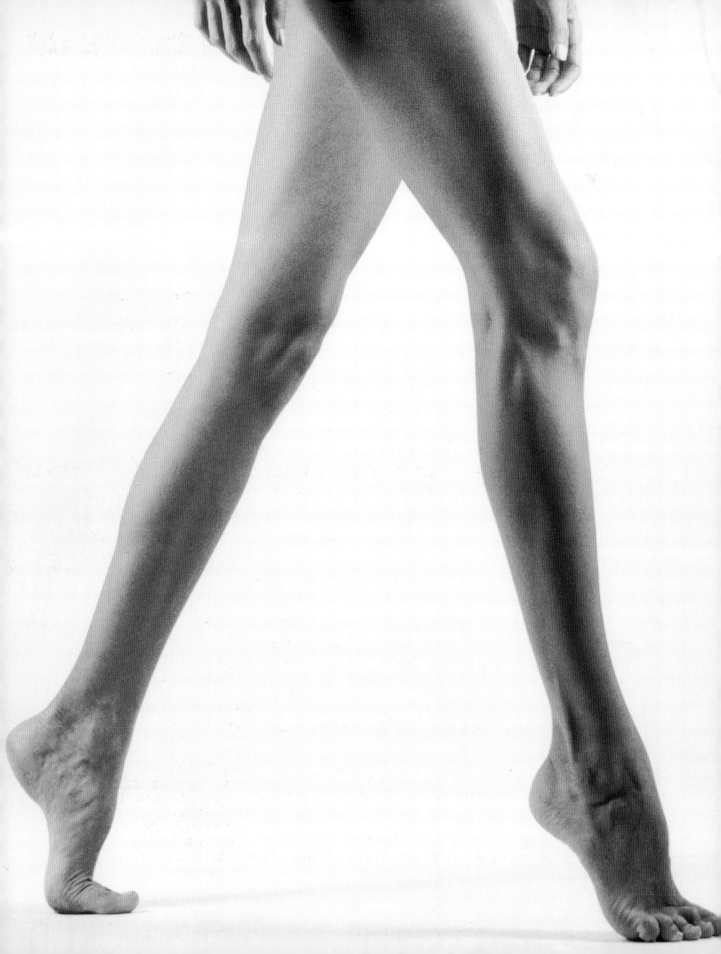

Legs take a stand

Pillars of femininity, columns of the temple …
The superlatives that legs attract set the bar very high—
and all the higher when hemlines are on the rise!

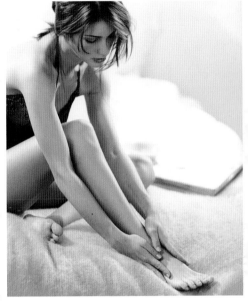

LEGGING IT

Models of fine architecture, our legs are the body's locomotives. The **thigh**, attached to the pelvis via the hip by the neck of the femur bone, benefits from an incredibly effective bundle of muscles (the quadriceps, adductors and hamstrings at the back). It continues into the **knee**, which is itself joined to the **calf** (containing the tibia and fibula bones), then the ankle.

SLENDER THIGHS, SHAPELY CALVES AND NARROW ANKLES

A supermodel's 1.12 m long legs are certainly out of reach unless you were born with them. The tyranny of the elongated thigh, flawless knee and fine ankle calls out for miracles. Fortunately, there's no lack of resources:

• protecting and **fluid-draining plants** (ginkgo biloba, red grape vine, cypress, sweet clover, dandelion).

• **anti-cellulite preparations** are increasingly clever and pleasurable to apply: use them to massage your legs, moving from the balls of the feet, the ankles, the back of the calf (essential) and the thighs, using circular movements, up to the hips and buttocks.

• the best activities: **walking**, **bicycle riding**, **barre exercises**.

GOOD NEWS

• support stockings now come in stay-up versions.

• there are very flattering self-tanning solutions available throughout the year.

• if you've got the shape for it, you can give yourself an extra 10 cm of curves with high heels (with the evening massage, page 180)!▶

Leg enemies
• A sedentary lifestyle
• Standing
• Excess weight
• Excess heat (watch out for baths!)
• Over-tight clothing

THE WORD FROM THE COACH
THIGH-SLIMMING PROGRAM
Standing up, knees straight, feet apart, pull in the stomach, squeeze the buttocks and stretch the left leg out, toes pointed, towards the front. Hold 2 seconds and rest (x 25 for each leg).

THE DETAILS IN CLOSE-UP

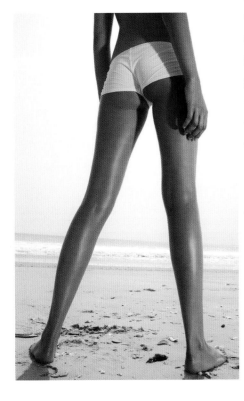

▶ **SECRETS FOR FIGHTING HEAVY LEGS**

• in the evening, finish off your bathroom routine with a **cold shower**, moving up the body from the calves to the thighs. Very effective against dilated veins and for washing away fatigue.

• a little massage with a special leg gel, cooled in the fridge to enhance the freshening effect and lathered on with your **feet up the wall** (legs vertical, at right angles to the back flat on the ground) for about ten minutes.

• in emergencies: massage the legs and thighs from bottom to top using a mixture based on menthol and camphor combined with an ingredient that stimulates the circulation.

• **sleep with your feet slightly elevated**, by slipping a leg-elevator under the ankles or a cushion under the mattress.

ADVICE FROM DR CLAUDE GARDE, ANGIOLOGIST

Circulation: keep it moving The movements and contractions of the muscles (the pressure of the heel on the ground, but also at the centre of the calves, where the blood is pushed) naturally propel the blood towards the heart. This is the 'venous return' – the 'backflow' of the blood, a dynamic facilitated by the valves in the veins of the legs that prevent the blood from going back downwards. Standing upright and immobile for too long hampers the process. If the system breaks down, it's called 'venous insufficiency'. The symptoms are: swollen ankles, tingling sensations, excessive cramps, but also spider veins, varicose veins and phlebitis (vein inflammation).

THE WORD FROM THE ANGIOLOGIST (a doctor specialising in the vascular system). The treatment of spider veins can't be undertaken before ensuring through further examination (a Doppler ultrasound) that there aren't any underlying varicose veins: untreated, a varicose vein can leave permanent marks. A phlebectomy, endovascular laser therapy or cryo-therapy may be performed.

For varicose veins

• **sclerotherapy**: an irritant is injected and the walls of the vein react by shrinking, disappearing in a few months. The **foam** version of the therapy is more effective on larger veins and reduces the number of sessions needed for smaller spider veins.

For spider veins

• **microsclerotherapy** applied to the small blood vessels: gentler products, finer needles. No immediate result either.

• **vascular lasers**: two kinds of laser act on differently coloured spider veins: from red (surface veins) to purple and blue ones (deep).

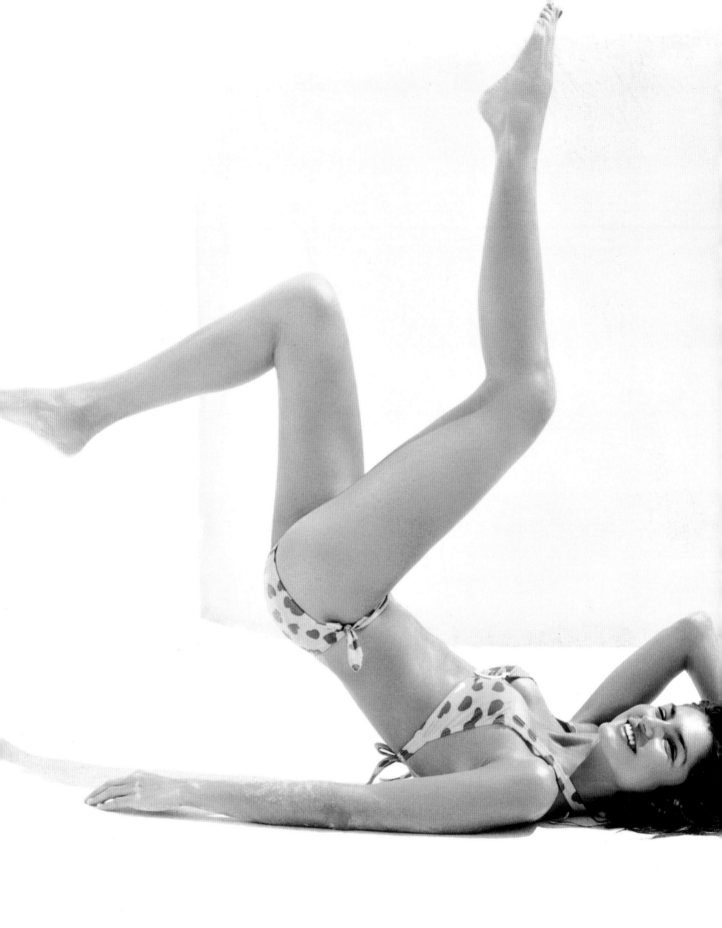

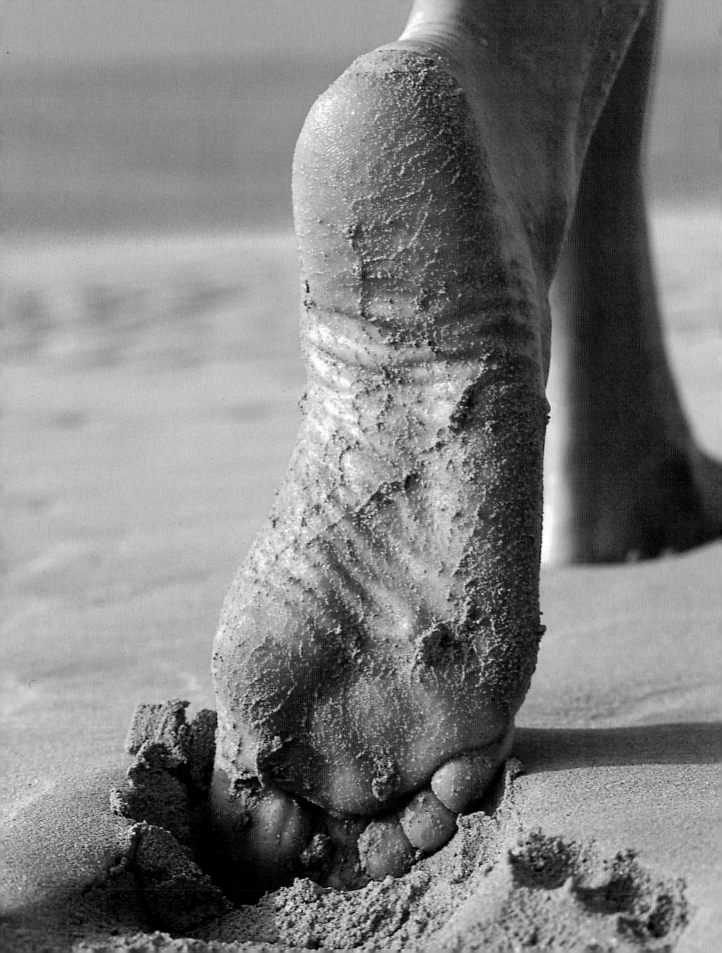

The world at my feet

They offer unlimited support (and transport).
Advice on the basics from podiatrist
Ari Darmon, so we can put our best foot forward ... bliss!

ORGANS IN THEIR OWN RIGHT, the feet valiantly carry the body's weight (multiplied by two or three when running!), on their **26 bones**, articulated in a cunning arrangement of muscles and tendons, to keep us stable. They are separated from the ground by a shock-absorbing pad. Under pressure, **hyperkeratosis** offers protection in the form of corns, calluses and other kinds of hard, thick skin. The **soles of the feet** and the palms of the hands are the only areas of skin without hair.

FLAT OR HIGH-ARCHED FEET?

If your shoe size is 38, the arch of the foot is on average 3.8 cm from the ground (4.1 cm for size 41). Above that and it is a high-arched foot; below, it is flat—which is the case for 80% of us. The big toe once was an opposable thumb that was rearranged.

THE NAILS, like those on the hands, are part of the **integumentary** system and need to be fed: the blood has to go the furthest to reach them, so they are the last served. When **circulation** is poor (especially in the legs), they become ridged and brittle.

THE SHOE supports the whole apparatus, hence the importance of choosing well, according to the shape of your foot and the use you'll be making of them—balancing style and functionality:

it's not normal to have pain!

THE SHAPE! Egyptian (a longer big toe), **Roman** (square, with the first three toes the same length) or **Greek** (a longer second toe).

The shape of the foot only makes a difference if you wear bad shoes, which can lead to corns, calluses, bunions and other deformities. The only response: see the podiatrist!

Once a week (but no more than that, heating stimulates calluses)
• rasp, pumice, then a gentle exfoliating scrub.

Every day After the shower or bath, you need something rich to moisturise, so add cream, cream and more cream! As a constant source of support, the foot needs to be as elastic as possible.

In the kit
• nail pliers (without going too far into the corners) and nail clippers
• cuticle pliers—tearing forbidden!
• nail file
• nail buffer
• moisturising cream.

THE WORD FROM THE PODIATRIST Walk barefoot on sand: this is one of best sole-massaging exercises; it finally lets each joint move freely.

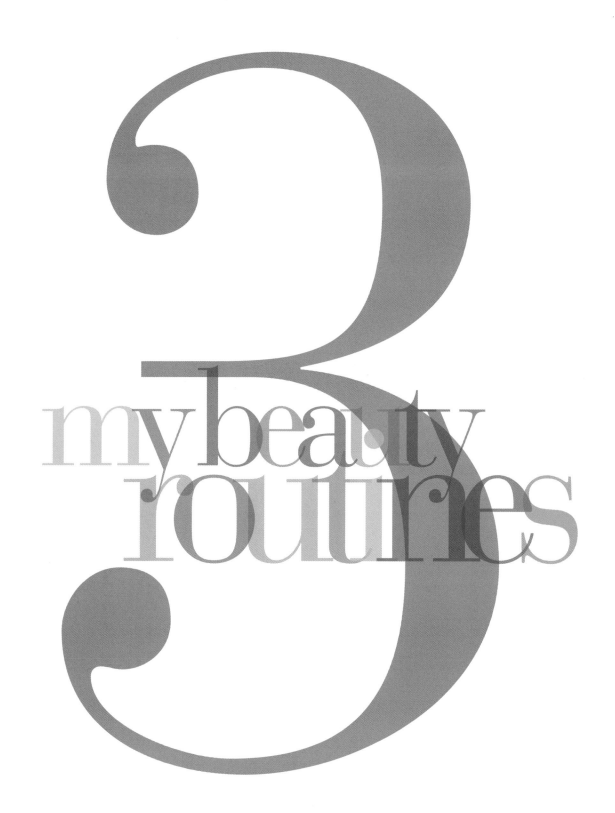

3

my beauty routines

PREFERENTIAL TREATMENTS

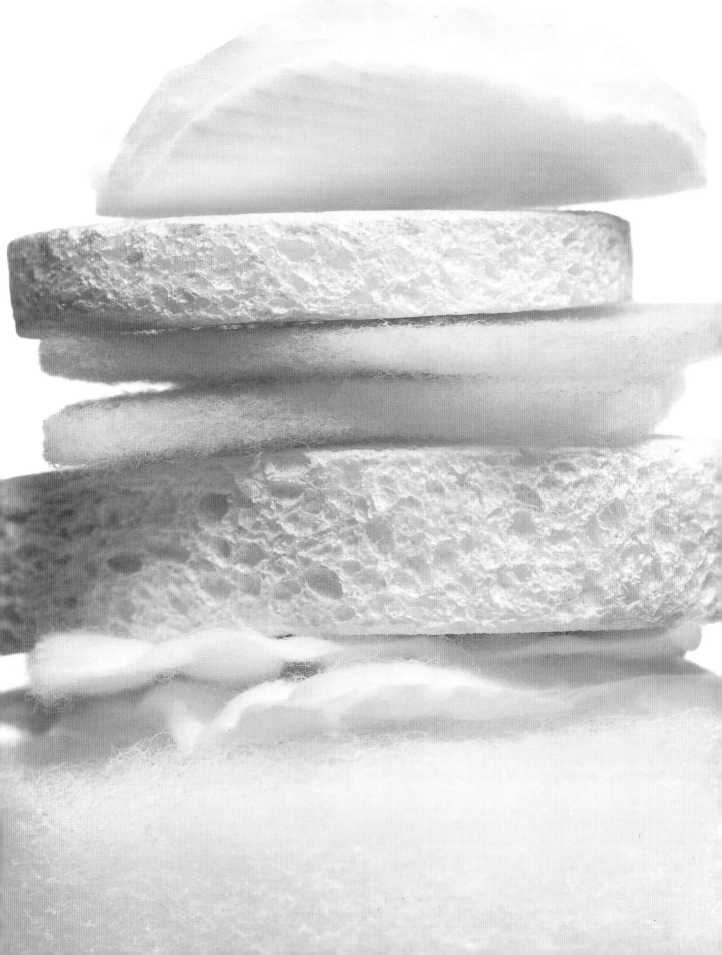

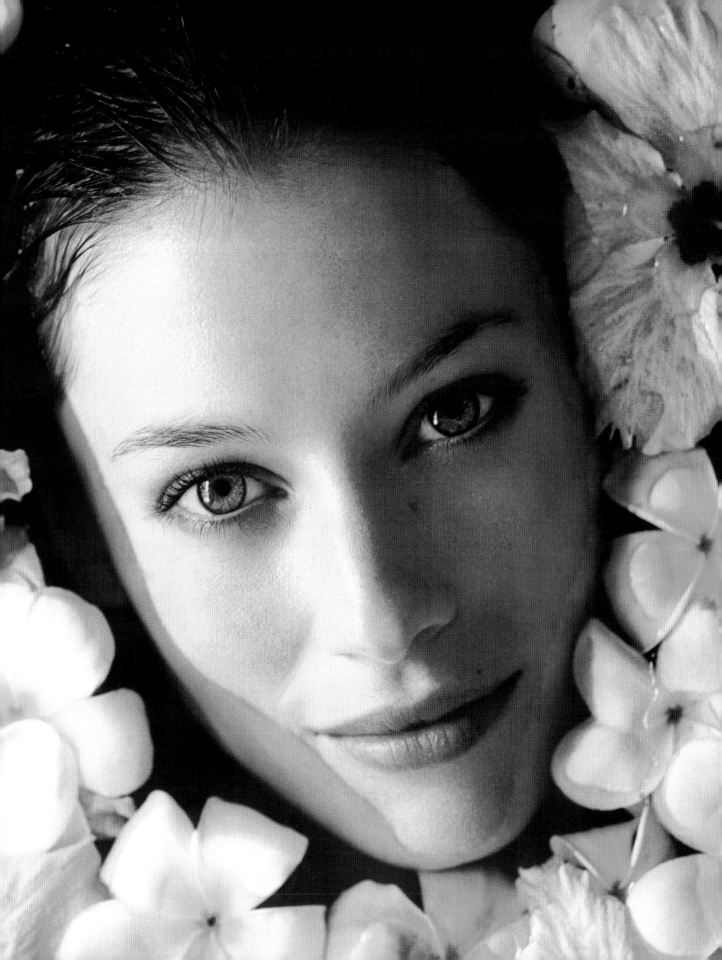

Facial care: beauty face to face

Freshness
on the menu

For a fresh start, wake up your skin properly and brighten your day. Professional advice for setting the right (skin) tone.

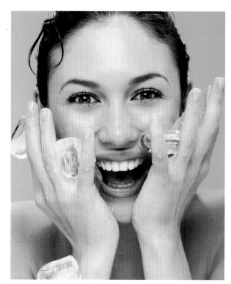

WAKE UP A 'MORNING FACE': JUST ADD WATER... AND OXYGEN

The one way to prepare the skin for any lotions and make-up? A thorough cleansing to get rid of all the night's debris ... and start out on the right foot!

Drink a large glass of mineral water on waking, then 30 seconds on the clock to wash away the traces of sleep and stimulate the **microcirculation** on the face and décolletage.

Start with tepid water, then move gradually to cold. For an energetic version, use the **shower**; for a gentler version, use cotton wool. In either case, wipe down the face well using a tissue to avoid dehydration.

A cotton bud dipped in lotion or water to **clean** any secretions from the night from the inside edge of the eye, then careful cleaning of the eyelashes to properly separate them, avoid clumping and rid them of any last traces of mascara.

Warm your day cream in your hand and **massage** the face, neck and décolletage, working outwards from the centre. A little extra dab around the eyes and mouth, smoothing out gently.

Remember to remove any excess cream before applying make-up, otherwise it won't hold.

As for **rosy cheeks**, you'll get them (almost) naturally: you just have to bring them out by giving your cheeks a light pinch.

THE MAKE-UP ARTIST'S SECRET
Applying ice directly to the skin, like in the photo, is out of the question (it burns!). But an ice cube in a face washer or towel works miracles on the freshness of the complexion!

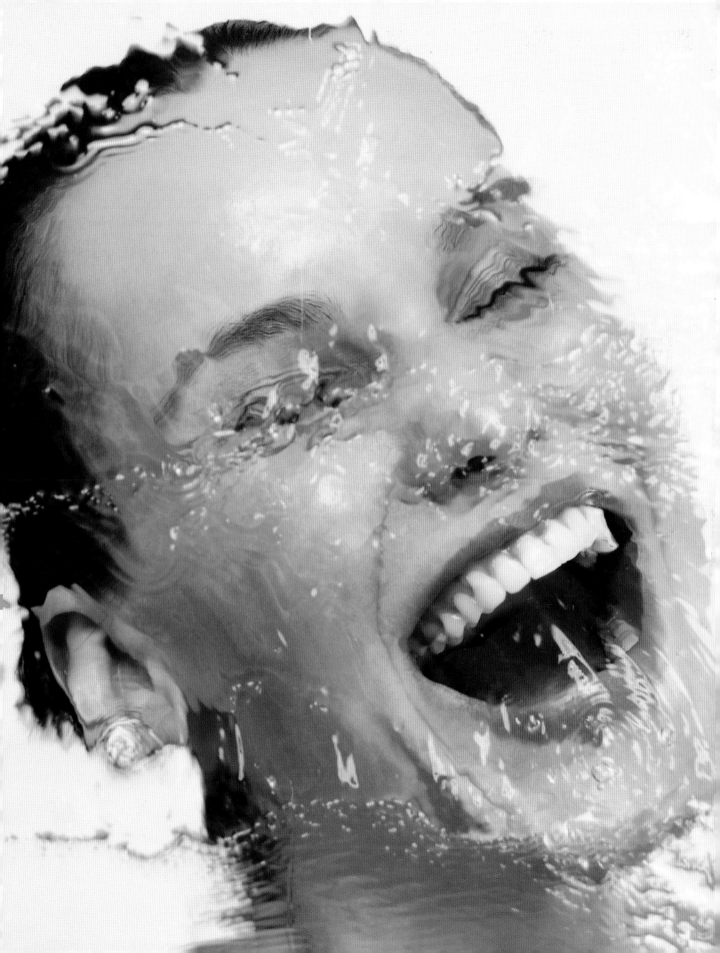

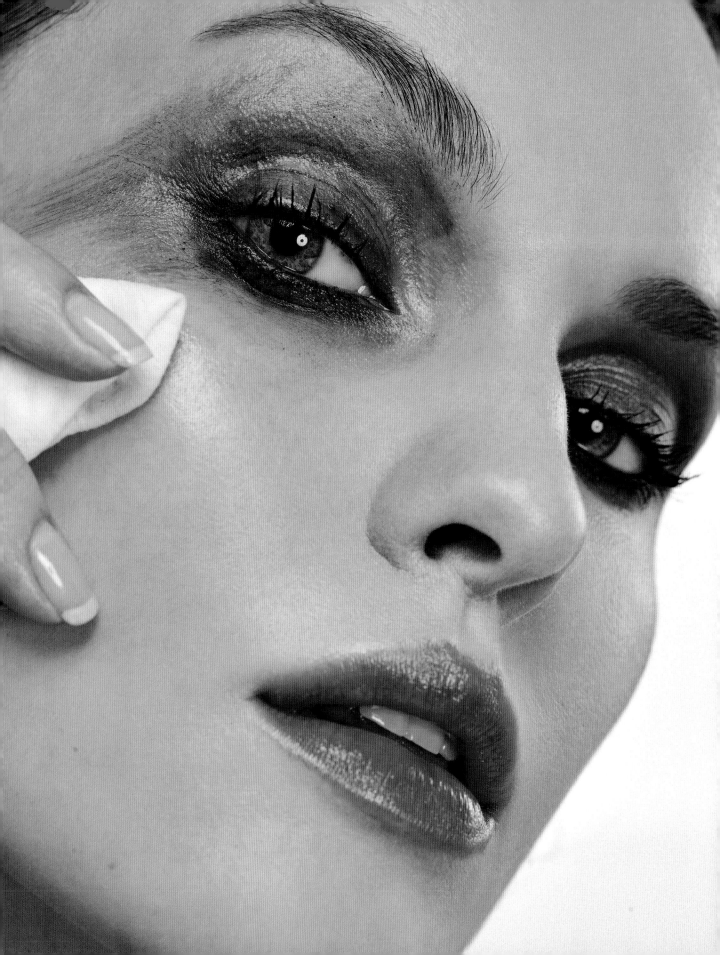

Around the eye
in the blink of an eye

Especially sensitive, the skin of the eyelids really deserves its own separate treatment ...

LOOK OUT: FRAGILE ZONE

The skin of the eyelids is extraordinarily fine and unimaginably complex: it has no fewer than seven layers, which multiplies the risks of swelling and other forms of pouching—the eye resting on a small pad of fat which can easily get out of shape. Perpetually moving muscles lead to the first wrinkles and fine lines.

ONLY CUSTOM-MADE

Products specifically designed for the area around the eye (anti-wrinkle, anti-shadow, anti-bag, anti-sag), ophthalmologically tested and tailored to its special sensitivity, are preferable to products made for the rest of the face, whatever their other qualities. The same principle applies to make-up removing creams and milks.

THE ART OF APPLICATION

Always using small quantities, and with infinite gentleness, dab on a little product and massage in, always using circular, clockwise movements. **Anti-shadow**, **anti-bag** treatments use fingertip pressure to drain by gently massaging from the outside towards the inside of the eye to boost the lymphatic system and drain fluid trapped inside the tissues.

UNMAKE-UP ME

Remove contact lenses (if you wear them!) • put a small amount of product on a make-up removing pad • place it against the eye area for a few seconds without rubbing to completely saturate the skin with product • wipe the pad towards the temples until no trace of make-up remains.

THE WORD FROM THE DERMATOLOGIST

EYE GYM: regularly pinch the skin from the root of the eyebrow to the temple to stimulate the upper eyelid, which has a tendency to droop.

OUT OF CIRCULATION only one out of three blood vessels work in this zone.

ADVICE FROM THE BEAUTICIAN

Oil-impregnated pads are still unbeatable for removing all traces of waterproof make-up.

Make-up removal
strictly speaking

*It's tempting, sometimes, to go to bed without removing make-up ...
But this is a bit like sleeping with all your clothes still on.
Take just a few minutes and your skin will thank you for it!*

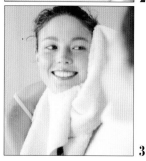

1

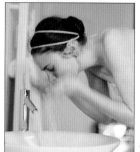

2

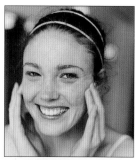

3

I'M CLEANING UP!

Before going to bed, removing make-up should be a priority: put everything else aside and diligently remove impurities, the dust left by all kinds of pollution, and excess sebum, to (finally) allow the skin to breathe.

Without daily make-up removal, the excess sebum may lead to the development of blocked pores (comedones), **the skin suffocates** and this accelerates the appearance of wrinkles. Nor is it any use applying a night cream to skin that hasn't been cleaned beforehand.

ALL THE FORMULAS

Even the classic make-up removing duo of **lotion and milk** now continue the work of daytime treatments by being adapted to your skin type. Another option, to be applied lavishly, are **foaming gels for rinsing off** using water, followed by careful drying (see images **1**, **2** and **3**).

Towelettes with gentle hypoallergenic **cleansing fluid** are ultra-practical.

ADVICE FROM THE DERMATOLOGIST
Water is not your skin's friend, especially if it tends to be dry or sensitive. There are now many no-rinse formulas, or products that can be simply removed with cotton wool.

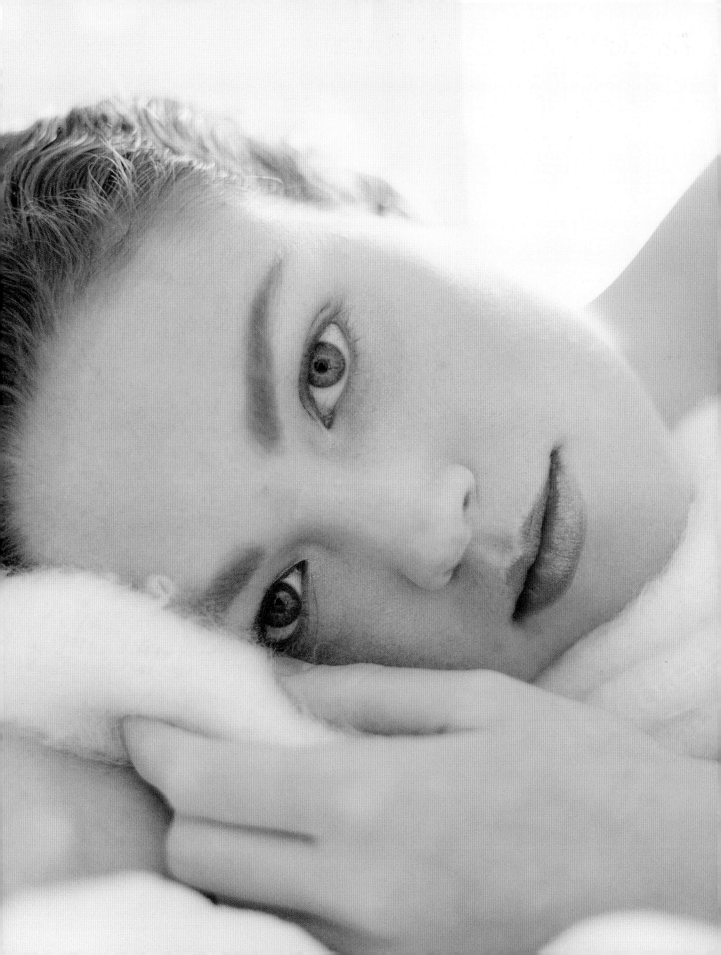

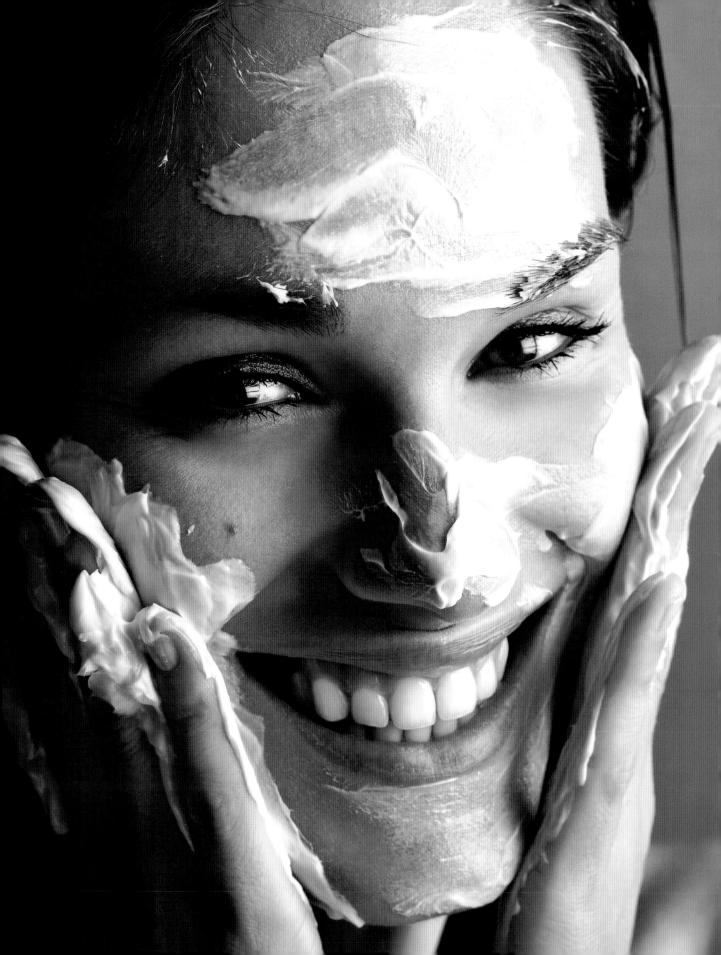

Hydration
quench your thirst

Water gives our skin its suppleness and elasticity—
it's our best passport to beauty.
The only problem: it's always trying to escape!

BEAUTY ELIXIR

Our skin contains on average 30% of all the water in our body … almost 9 litres! And yet, our body has to work daily to prevent this water—which is our No 1 guarantee of beautiful skin—from escaping. The process of hydration, which also enables toxins to be eliminated, follows an extremely delicate irrigation circuit which moves through all of the inner layers and regulates the evaporation of this water on the surface. The **stratum corneum** effectively reinforces its security measures thanks to **NMF**s **(natural moisturising factors)**, which trap water and distribute it or keep it in reserve according to the temperature.

The signs of dehydration (when the moisture threshold drops from 13% water in a normally hydrated epidermis to 10%): The skin feels tight, appears dull … The ultimate test: when you get up in the morning your skin holds the crease of the pillow. No doubt about it: your skin is thirsty!

HYDRATION, THE MAJOR BEAUTY MOVE

Hydration treatments will arrest the evaporation of moisture while helping the epidermis to knit its hydrolipidic film together and strengthen its barrier function. Choose according to your skin type, with star-performer active ingredients (glycerin, urea, ammonium lactate …).

Drink up!
The rule of at least 1.5 litres water a day (2 litres when hot) still applies!

THE WORD FROM THE DERMATOLOGIST
ATOMISERS: HOW THEY WORK
Spraying the face with spring or mineral water doesn't only have a deliciously refreshing effect: it helps to mechanically rebuild the hydrolipidic film by preventing drying. The sprayed water evaporates instead of the moisture from the epidermis … The moisture that impregnates the stratum corneum comes mainly from the dermis and gradually evaporates: 'useless' perspiration represents 20% of our daily water loss.

Nourish
day after day

Rejuvenate your skin in a few minutes:
freshness routines that transform the everyday!

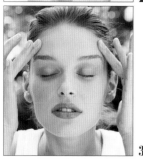

1

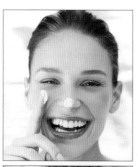

2

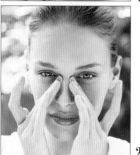

3

GOURMET CARE IN 3 ACTS!

1 **CHOOSE** the right formula: the one whose texture gives you pleasure and whose fragrance (or lack of fragrance) appeals, in addition to the specific benefit connected to your skin type.

2 **DRAIN** Apply light pressure with your fingertips to decongest the critical zones around the eyes at the root of the eyebrows.

3 **SMOOTH** the features, moving upwards. The skin is able to appreciate the care given to it by sending the right messages to the brain.

Night creams: for skin that tends to be dry, use rich creams with an oil-in-water texture.

Day creams: light, water-in-oil formulas.

ADVICE FROM THE BEAUTICIAN
Face massage is extraordinarily relaxing and will gently stimulate the blood and lymphatic microcirculation. And it reinforces the active ingredients of the products you use to an amazing extent.

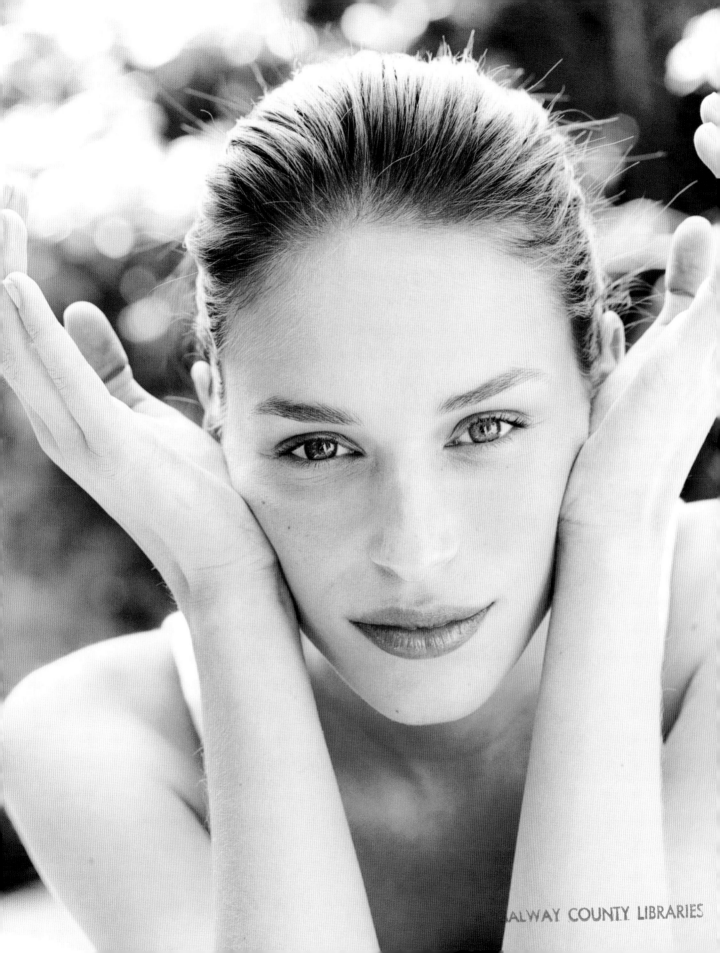

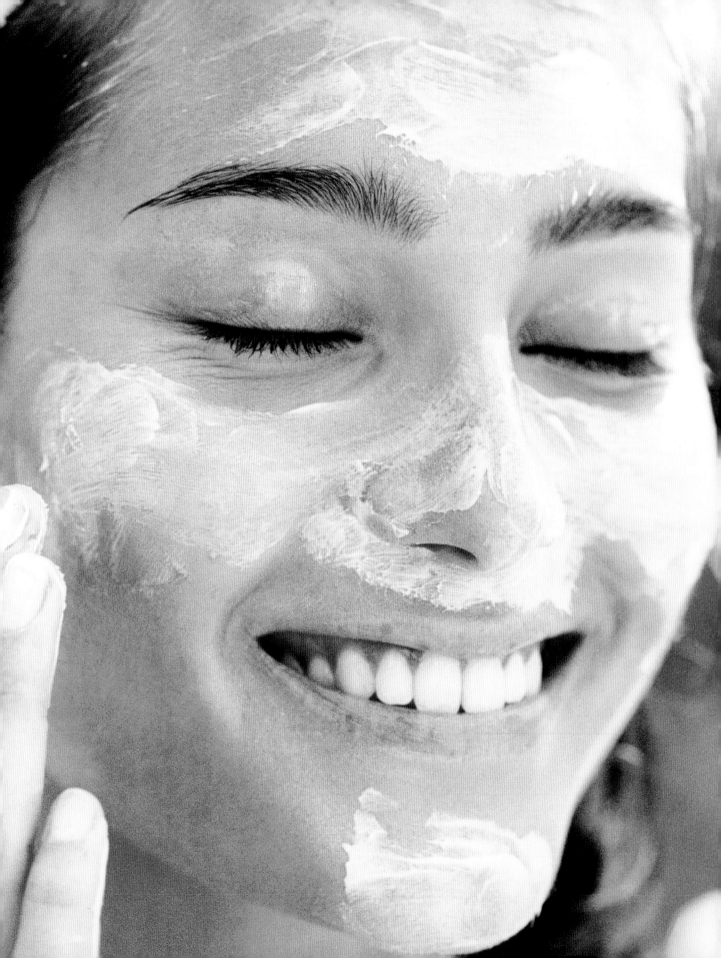

Exfoliation
radiance is mine!

Do something for your skin: purifying masks that deep-clean the face and let it receive the full benefit of the special treatment you lavish on it.

MAD FOR EXFOLIATION!

During exfoliation the stimulation of the face's microcirculation brightens the complexion, readying it to respond gratefully to active ingredients. On completely clean and make-up-free skin, apply the exfoliant and gently massage using small circular movements, including around the mouth, neck and décolletage (but avoiding the area around the eyes). Do this weekly.

HOME PEELS AND MICRO-DERMABRASION

Mild dermabrasion formulas, which offer the luxury of a professional treatment, using fruit extracts for a mini-peel.

BEAUTY MASKS

- **cleansing**: cleans and exfoliates, eliminates impurities and dead skin cells.
- **oily skin balancing**: absorbs excess sebum and normalises the pH balance.
- **hydrating**: moistens and boosts the hydration process to repair the hydrolipidic film.
- **firming**: stimulates the tissues through vasodilation (dilating the blood vessels).
- **lifting**: skin-tensing ingredients with a smoothing effect.

BRIGHT EYES

- ultra-gentle facial exfoliator • use delicate circular movements all around the eyes to rid your eye area of dead skin cell debris
- dab your eyes with an eye cream or mineral water • apply an anti-ageing mask especially designed for the fragile area around the eyes.

Pure clay the unsurpassed classic of cleansing masks. **THE WORD FROM THE DERMATOLOGIST** Creams based on vitamins E and C— top-ranking star ingredients—brighten the complexion.

UV rays
taming the sun

Strengthening your skin's natural defences so you only get the sun's benefits: just a fairytale? No, it's real—as long as a few myths are debunked.

THE GOLDEN RULES FOR SAFE TANNING

• **prepare yourself** from the inside (melanin boosters to improve the skin's tolerance) at least ten days beforehand … and during.

• **sunbathe less** … and never between 10 a.m. and 4 p.m. (even underneath an umbrella).

• **check** your skin phototype (page 19) by asking yourself this question: 'Do I burn before tanning or not?', but be conservative in any case with your skin's natural reserves, some of which are spent with each exposure.

• the **SPF** factor (sun protection factor against UVA and UVB rays) enables you to assess the level of physical and chemical protection (against sunburn) and also on the internal level (against cell damage).

• **choose** products with high protection ratings, opting, especially at the beginning, for 30+ products.

• **cover yourself** with sunscreen from head to foot, but without rubbing it in too much so that the filters stay on the surface and don't lose their effectiveness, use a high-protection stick for delicate areas, and **reapply every 2 hours**, whatever the rating.

• **'water resistant'** = two 20-minute dips 15 minutes apart. Except that drying yourself off after each dip (essential so that you don't turn yourself into a magnifying glass) means you need to reapply.

• **compound** the benefits with anti-age, anti-dehydration, firming, anti-sensitivity, slimming or oil-regulating formulas (to avoid nasty surprises when you get home). And keep your usual day cream (to be applied in the morning before sun-exposure), if it doesn't come in a version with sunscreen.

No moderation required
As a complement to your sun protection: self-tanning products, bronzing powders, luminisers and beauty oils add sunshine to your spirits from the first days.

Sun therapy
The visible rays of the sun are champion antidepressants and stress-busters.

THE WORD FROM THE DOCTOR
The sun sets the calcium in the bones, thanks to the synthesis of vitamin D, a vital process which also prevents osteoporosis. Minimum recommended dose for an adult: 15 minutes a day.

THE RIGHT FACTOR
What level of protection?
• 4: low
• 8: medium
• 15+: high
• 30+: very high.

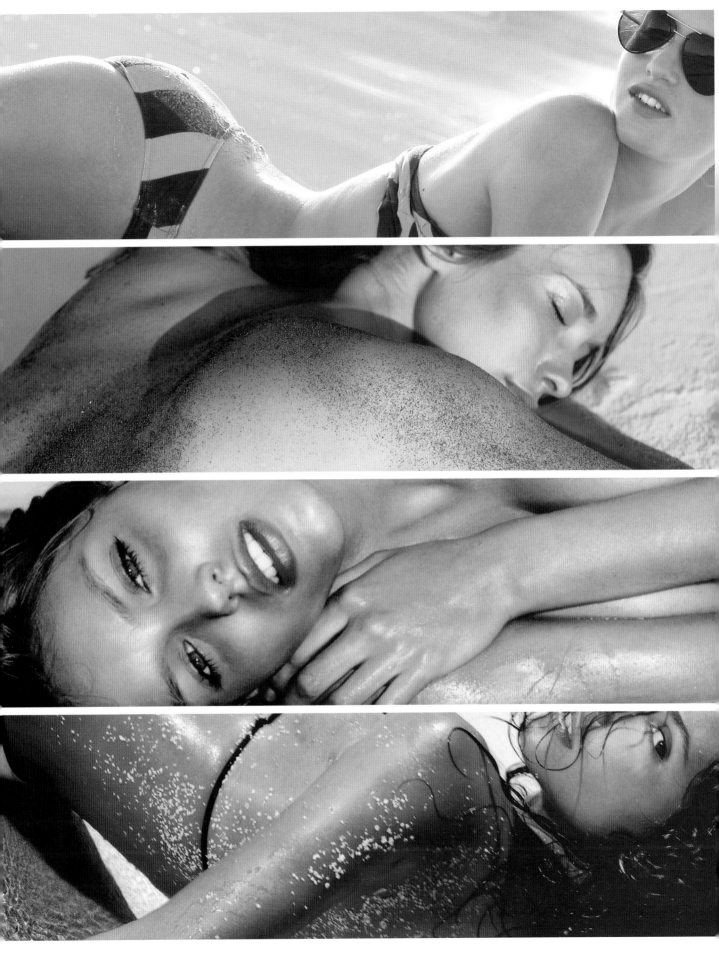

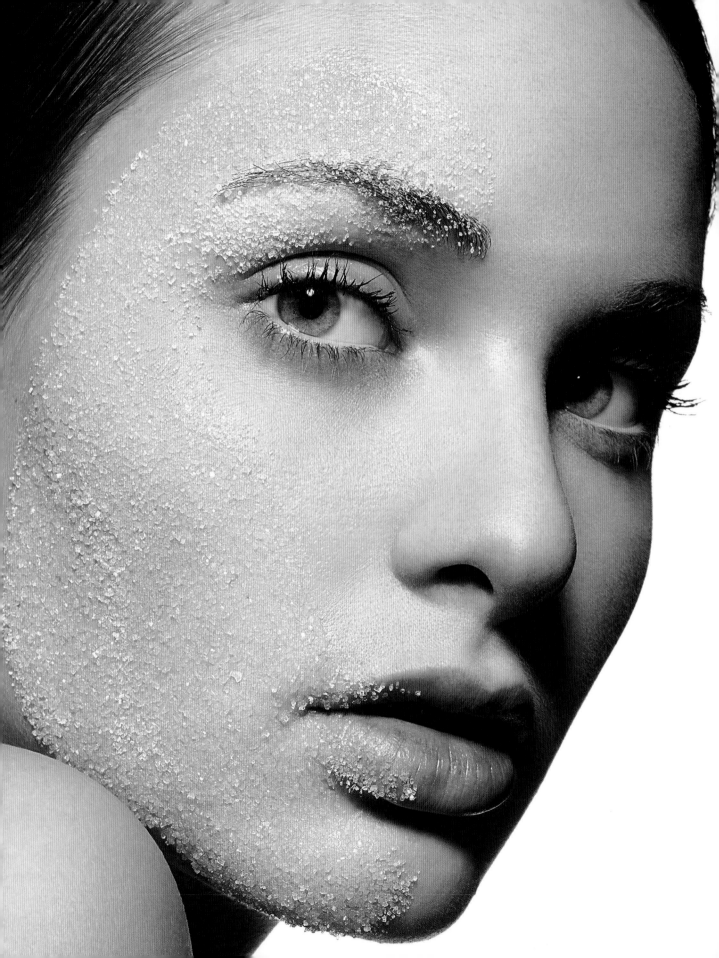

Anti-irritation
actions against reactions

With the weather and UV rays, our skin lives under constant attack.
With special formulas for sensitive and reactive skins or
anti-pollution products, cosmetic treatments come to the rescue …

Cold, fatigue, sun, heat, stress, pollution, tap water and unsuitable cosmetics: these are, in decreasing order of aggressiveness, the troublemakers identified by a study* commissioned by L'Oréal. Symptoms that are neurosensory in origin (inflammations, itching, tingling, redness) suggest to scientists the possibility of a neurophysiological mechanism governing skin sensitivity—clearly their causes are partly neurological. Some, like pollution (whose nasty effects can be seen on a simple make-up remover pad), have harmful consequences which are undeniably felt as soon as one finds onself in an urban environment.

AM I ALLERGY PRONE?

• **Sensitive or reactive skin**, my skin has a more intense reaction than a 'normal' skin to the same stimulus.

• **Intolerant skin** reacts very strongly to pollution, hard water, wind, cold and sun, and certain cosmetic or make-up products.

• **Atopic skin** has abnormally high levels of permeability: the stratum corneum is easily penetrated by any agent, whether an irritant or not.

• **Allergic skin**, my skin has developed a specific sensitivity to one or more external agents (immune reaction to allergens).

*Source: Ipsos Health & Beauty—France: panel 5134 women aged 12+

THE WORD FROM THE DERMATOLOGIST
One more reason to stop smoking? Tobacco is a misogynist! It has an even greater effect on female skin, bringing out in an even more dramatic way the visible signs of smoking (wrinkles around the mouth and eyes, vertical folds on the cheeks, muddy complexion). Not forgetting the nicotine that settles in the pores and blackens comedones by oxidising them.

ADVICE FROM THE EXPERT : SENSITIVE SKIN

Dr Pascale Mathelier-Fusade
Dermatologist and allergist

Attached to the allergy clinic of Tenon Hospital in Paris, at the cutting edge of research on sensitive and reactive skin, Dr Pascale Mathelier-Fusade is now working with sensitive skin specialists Mixa, which has set the standard in skin protection for the last forty years.

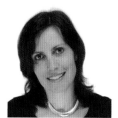

'The fact that we constantly require our skin to adapt runs the risk of weakening it!'

SENSITIVE SKIN IS SPREADING!

An effect of fashion or the result of our more aggressive environment? Whatever the causes, more and more women are reporting they have sensitive skin … It's not easy an easy phenomenon to define—for a long time it was described as 'fragile' skin, because of its subjective element. It's not easy to quantify a feeling of tightness, tingling and burning sensations, even if there are objective parameters available. Very fine skin that flushes at the least emotion; dry skins that don't seem to be able to tolerate any cosmetic product; naturally intolerant skins, very fine, often suffering from mild rosacea. But more and more of my patients have skin that was not originally sensitive—it has been weakened following localised skin treatments (anti-acne treatments, inappropriate or excessive exfoliation). This hypersensitivity is the result of damage to the skin barrier, or stratum corneum, the uppermost surface layer, infinitely delicate, that is the hydrolipidic film.

THE SKIN'S MAIN ENEMIES?

WATER is the No 1 aggressor: hard or not, mineral or not, it comes in just ahead of detergents (**soaps, cleansing gels**). This has been extensively demonstrated in the case of the hands; it is also true for the face.

Changes in climate, exposure to the sun or excessive cold are also culprits. Not only is cold a threat in itself, but the skin suffers from swings in temperature. When we move from a cold to a warm environment, the blood vessels dilate easily. On the face, where the network of blood vessels is so delicate, the flushing that results can persist for several minutes. Similarly, air conditioning has a damaging effect on the skin by drying it out.

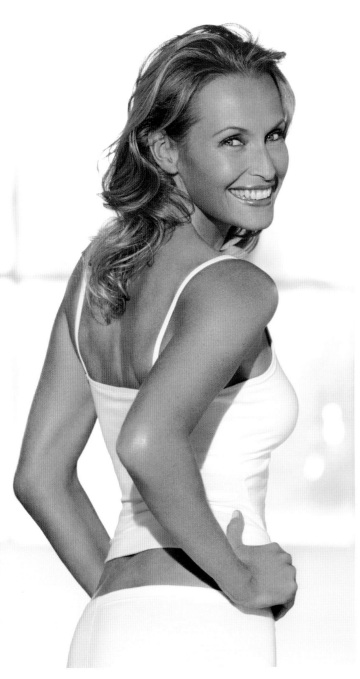

People who are hyper-reactive, whose nose and eyes react to all of these factors, certainly know about it. **Pollution** is also obviously an aggravating factor.

'SENSITIVE SKIN': INCONVENIENCE OR ILLNESS?

AT WHAT POINT DO WE CALL IT AN ALLERGY?

What is the difference between allergy and intolerance? When a woman can't tolerate anything any more and no product works for her, neither her day cream nor her night cream, she concludes: 'I must be allergic!' But it's more complicated than that! There's an easy way of differentiating an allergy and an intolerance: with an allergy, there's itching, scratching—eventually the skin flakes off; whereas sensitive (intolerant) skin, produces burning sensations, feelings of tightness, irritation, tingling …

How can this sensitivity be tested and what range of effects does it cover? An ever-more diverse range of effects, given that the analysis is based on subjective reports … We can say whether a product is allergenic, but when it comes to sensitivity, the only criteria for judging are what the patient says.

The skin is the mirror of the soul, even if the correlation between stress and sensitive skin hasn't been clearly established, except in the case of contact allergies—it has been proven that psoriasis and seborrheic dermatitis (which affects the scalp, eyebrows, nostril area) can be triggered by states of stress, but it's very difficult to isolate the trigger factors.

What is certain is that we spend our life adapting and developing an armour for resisting attack. The fact that we constantly require our skin to adapt runs the risk of weakening it …

ESTELLE LEFÉBURE, CHARM AMBASSADOR, is a perfect symbol of freshness and the values of Mixa, the sensitive skin specialists.

SENSITIVE SKIN

'Reactive skin is protected using barrier, soothing, nourishing formulas...'

What is the difference between sensitive and hypersensitive skin?

Sensitive skin doesn't tolerate certain products, whereas hypersensitive skin doesn't tolerate any!

Fair 'Caucasian'-type skin is at greater risk—Asiatic and dark skins, which are thicker, are in principle more protected. No skin type is safe—even combination skins can be affected. And the phenomenon more particularly affects women aged between 20 and 45. Later on, the focus is more on wrinkles and skin dryness.

Sensitive skin is not 'hereditary', but a genetic factor has been identified in certain cases, such as rosacea conditions.

Dry skin is dull, tight, uncomfortable—whereas very dry skin will go so far as to flake off.

Choosing products that are not only specifically adapted to your skin but don't require rinsing gives an extra measure of security and effectiveness.

THE DERMATOLOGIST'S ADVICE FOR SOOTHING SENSITIVE SKIN

WHEN IT COMES TO COSMETIC SOLUTIONS, HYDRATION IS THE KEY WORD.

AND THEN SOFTEN, NOURISH, SOOTHE...

For fine skins, stick to moisturising masks—and banish deep-cleansing or exfoliating masks, which are much too extreme.

PROTECT with 'barrier' formulas; use specifically adapted products that are soothing, nourishing, moisturising, limiting water use as much as possible.

The sun can provide relief by calming down feelings of tightness, but on the other hand it aggravates skin that tends to redness or rosacea, hence the need for protection.

AVOID EXFOLIATING: the consequences are worse than the benefits.

When it comes to **diet**, there are no particular prohibitions, but it is sensible to only consume moderate amounts of things that will contribute to the dilation of blood vessels: alcohol, spices, and eating or drinking things that are too hot …

Dr Pascale Mathelier-Fusade

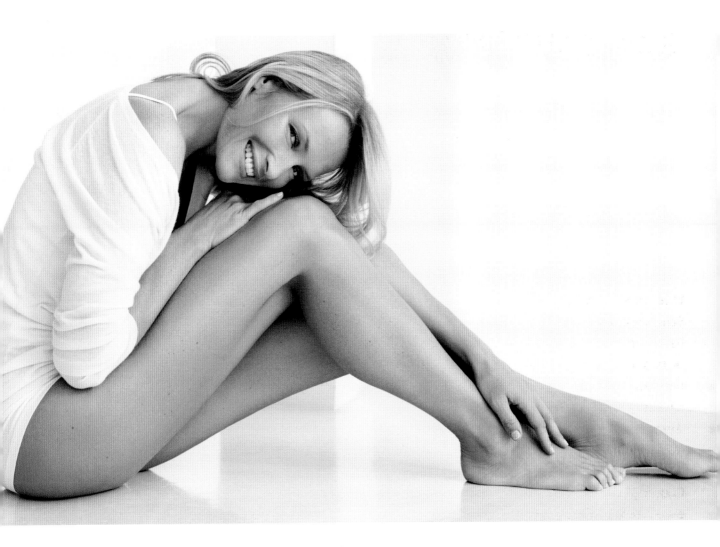

THE WORD FROM THE LAB:
HOW A PRODUCT EARNS THE HYPOALLERGENIC LABEL

We've had a policy of excellence for 45 years: taking care of the most fragile skins is no small challenge. The Mixa ethos produces **formulas under medical supervision, rigorously tested under the supervision of dermatologists**. Our charter is dedicated to the design of high-tolerance formulas, using a strict principle: a minimum number of ingredients (since multiplying the number of ingredients also multiplies the risk of allergy) selected for their innocuousness, in compliance with standards of optimum purity, demanding the complete traceability of all of the raw materials used. Each formula is analysed by a group of experts—dermatologists, toxicologists and pharmacologists—first in the laboratory, on 'reconstructed skin' (a patented L'Oréal technology), which mimics the real reactive process of the skin, then on live volunteers under the supervision of dermatologists using patch tests. If there is the least intolerance or irritation, the formula is abandoned. But Mixa sets the bar even higher: earning the hypoallergenic label (to minimise the risk of allergy in baby-product ranges and very sensible and reactive skins) makes this process even more demanding, with the number of patch tests being multiplied to measure the allergy-resistant ability of the skin, even under extreme conditions of use. It only takes a single dubious reaction for the formula to be rejected.

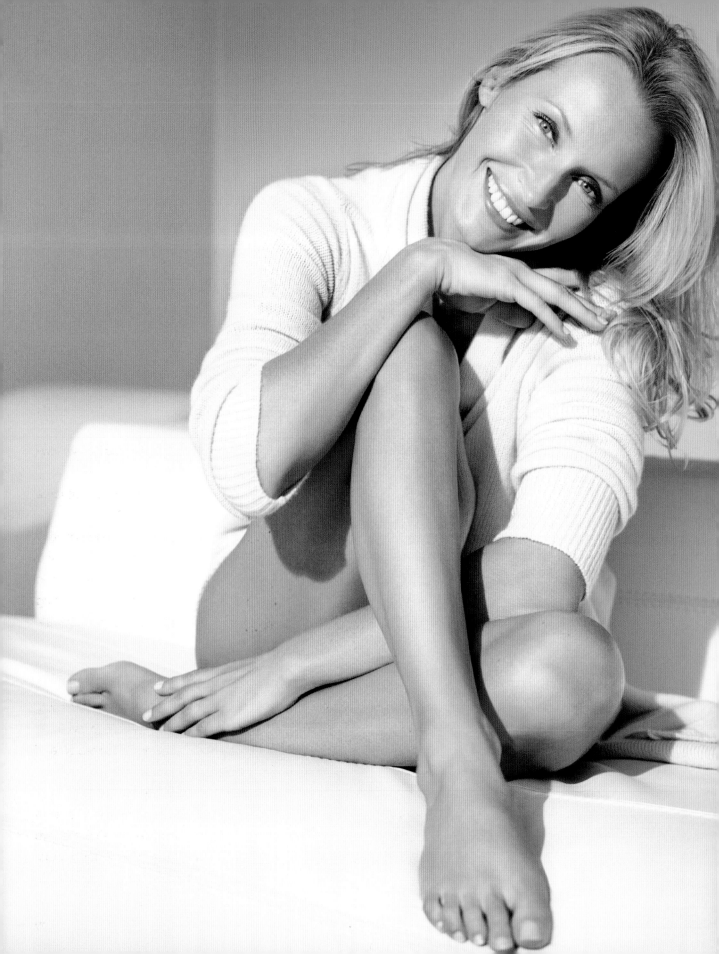

'Sensitivity, is something very fine, very soft—the senses are heightened!'

ESTELLE LEFÉBURE
TOP MODEL, ACTRESS … AND MOTHER

MY DEFINITION OF SENSITIVITY?

Sensitivity is a concept that is very powerful on a symbolic level, including very positive aspects. It's something very fine, very soft—the senses heightened …

It's sensing and feeling everything. Every gesture, every word, every vibration … including negative ones. Even if it's important to control our sensitivity, we all need it, we need to learn to cultivate it—it's a bit like the innocence left over from childhood, something of our virginity, something very pure, which can gradually be lost over the years.

My daughters are 12 and 10 years old. I try to make them sensitive to the simple things, so they keep their freshness—so they don't only react to 'extra-ordinary' things.

For several years I've been a spokesperson for the organisation *L'enfant bleu, enfance maltraitée* (which offers psychological support to abused children).

It's a form of engagement in the strongest sense, since these children are literally given a voice—a painful subject that moves me more than anything else. It's so poignant to see these children's drawings … I am also involved in programs for the education of young girls with *Marie Claire*, and in Africa, with UNICEF. So many causes that are close to my heart, as a mother and as a woman: being so well supported and pampered—I find it completely natural to give some of the wealth in my life back, without expecting anything in return.

MY BEAUTY ROUTINE

For me, this is always connected to a whole lifestyle … Each of us is given a certain amount of 'beauty capital'. To try to preserve it as best we can, beyond routines there are lifestyle rules to follow.

My golden rule: a good diet, lots of vegetables, very little meat and fish … I'm a very green tea type of person, it's my favourite drink, very organic, packed full of antioxidants.

I set aside little moments to give myself a total cleanse: **clean skin is an absolute** for me.

I wear very little makeup—I just pinch my cheeks for a blush effect. Above all I don't overdo it, even in the evening. A dab of gloss, a hint of shadow, a little mascara and pencilled eyebrows because they are fair, never any foundation, I just use concealer on the little imperfections and I use powder for photos.

'My younger daughter adores putting on cold cream, right in the middle of her cheeks, it's so cute!'

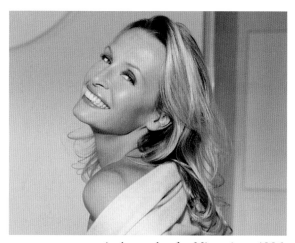

Ambassador for Mixa since 1996, Estelle's film career is also nothing to be sniffed at. In Le bal des actrices, *in which Maïwenn Le Besco pays homage to great French actresses, she finds her best role … as herself!*

I always make cleaning the skin a priority …
And, before going to bed, I have my little ritual: cream on my hands, balm around the lips, and water flavoured with ginger. From time to time, a moisturising or purifying mask. I take time out for a massage, or a more intense hydration treatment.

GOOD SPORT!

I do stretching exercises at the gym, I do a lot of horse riding—dressage. It's a real pleasure, not necessarily good for the back, but so helpful for the head!

I am a great believer in the habits you learn when you're very young. I teach my daughters routines to protect their skin, they adore the Mixa *bébé* cold cream—it's wonderful, they put some on in the morning. The youngest one puts a ring of it right in the middle of her cheeks, it's so cute! And at least I know that even with the cold and the pollution, her little cheeks are protected!

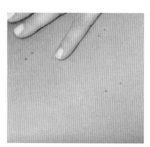 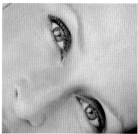 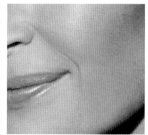 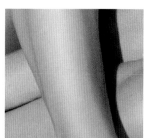

MORNING AND EVENING, A COMPLETE CLEANSE, but gently, with Soothing Cleansing Water (*Eau Démaquillante Apaisante*). I adore the fresh sensation of cleaning with water—and sometimes if I am coming from a shoot, I use a cleansing milk between two water cleanses.
DURING THE DAY, I am hooked on my Mixa *Effet Soleil* (Mixa Sun Effect) cream, it gives me a healthy look and it's very easy to apply. And the with the sun, I take a softly-softly approach, even if, paradoxically, my blonde skin gets used to it quickly.

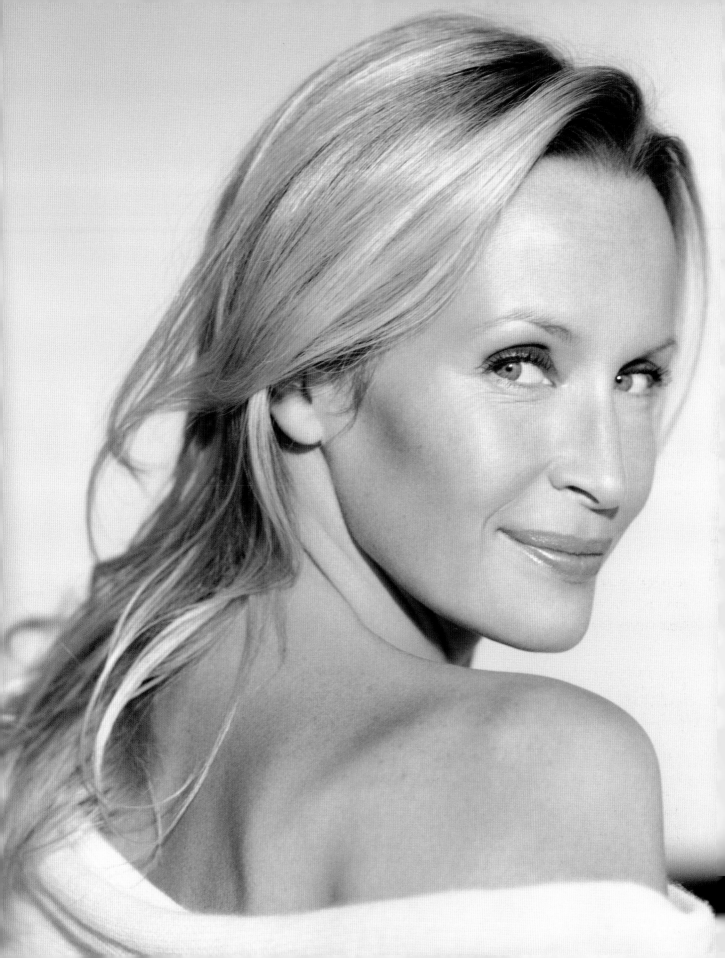

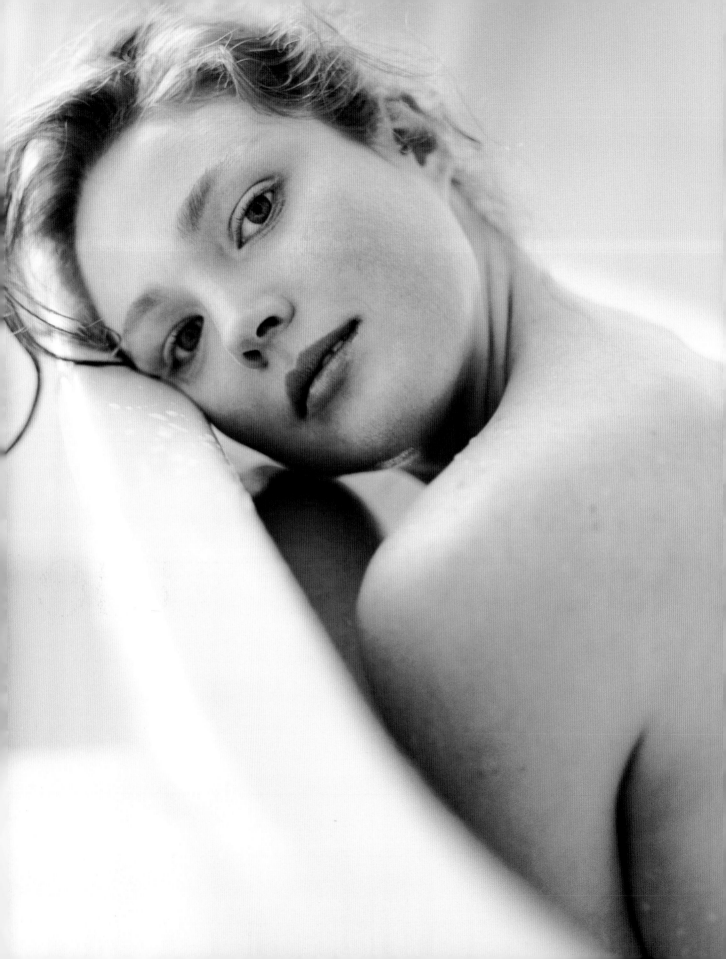

Self care: the body in tune

Baths
sink into serenity

*A moment of indulgence par excellence,
a bath is much more about relaxation than hygiene.
Good things to know before immersing yourself in its delights …*

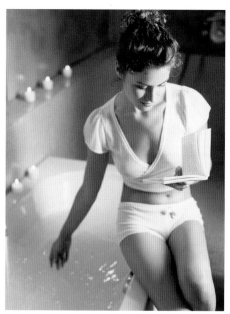

THE RIGHT TEMPERATURE

Even if a hot bath soothes muscle aches, it mustn't be too hot or it could stress the heart or have a disastrous effect on the veins in the legs. So, 37°C is the maximum temperature, and preferably 33°C, especially before bedtime (to lower the body temperature), leaving your legs out of the water (they love being raised) and ideally finishing off with a cool shower. **Essential oils** preserve the hydrolipidic film, while at same time offering you the multiple benefits of plants, seaweeds, minerals, relaxing or rejuvenating, slimming or purifying: we absorb them as much through the pores of our skin as through the fragrances they give off. This is also the ideal time for a **beauty mask**, or for **gently pumicing** the knees, elbows and feet.

TWENTY MINUTES OF WEIGHTLESSNESS

Leave behind the everyday by allowing yourself to float, a form of therapy that's extremely easy to practise at home. Set aside the necessary time, unplugging the telephone and chasing away unpleasant thoughts. A small inflatable cushion under the neck if the bathtub isn't ergonomically designed, back unknotted, knees loose, relax the jaw and let the soothing waves of endorphins flow over you.

Limit yourself to twenty minutes max, both to avoid getting a chill … and emerging all crumpled.

THE WORD FROM THE EXPERT
Create a bubble of relaxation, with perfumed candles, a good book and soft music.

To avoid extremes, it is sensible to limit your water heater's thermostat to 55°C.

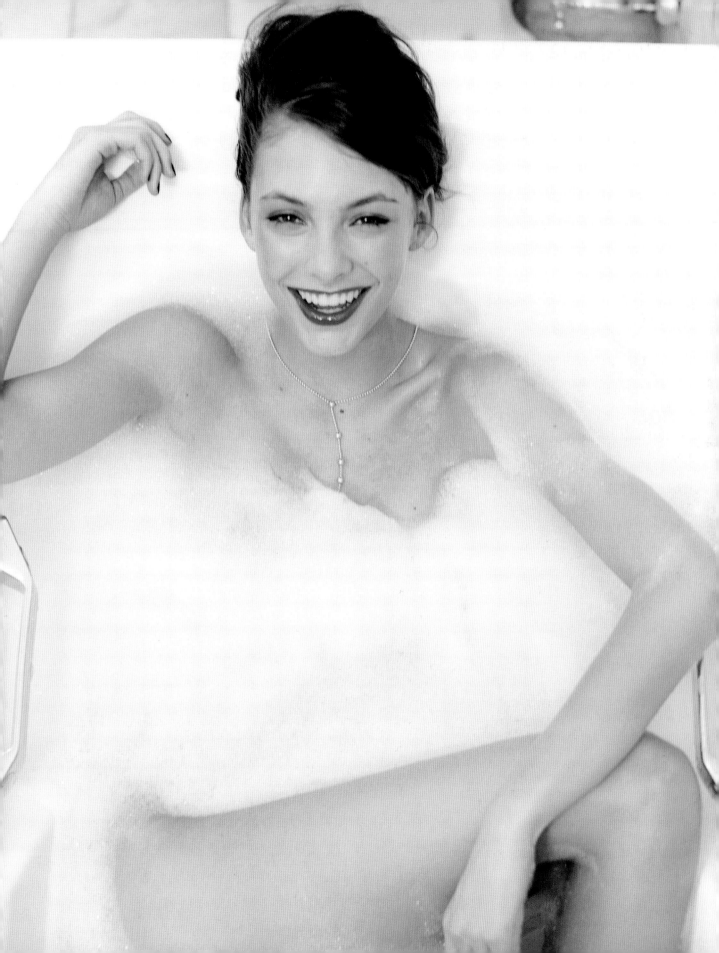

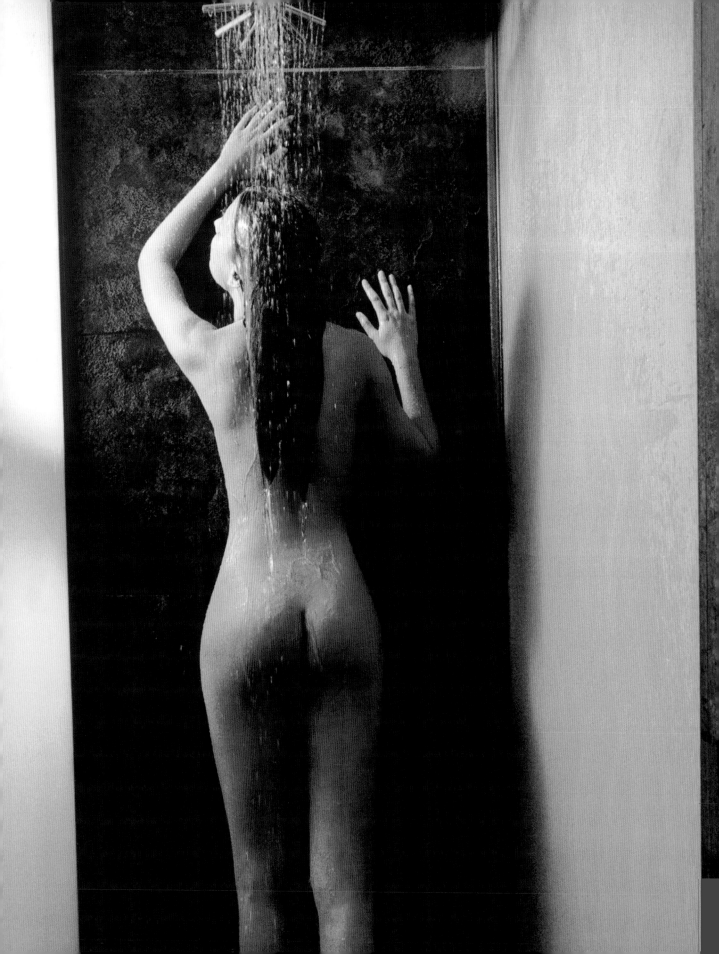

Shower power

The supreme tonic, it's able to reset the wake-up alarm, clear the mind, and wash away tiredness and stress. And, as a bonus, there's no more effective way of getting clean!

IN THE MORNING ... bonus tone-up!

It's the way to get rid of tensions resulting from a bad sleeping position, muscle spasms and other back troubles: pressure jets and well-directed streams can relax the muscles and provide the crack of the whip needed to restart a machine still in nocturnal sleep mode.

AT THE END OF THE DAY

Summer ... it gets rid of sweat, sand and salt, coming back from the beach or a hike, or the debris from a city scorcher. Particularly beneficial and relaxing, it lets the body forget the heat of the day and gives relief to the legs (as long as the final jet of water is cold).

Winter ... it washes away pollution and built-up fatigue, and lets you recharge your batteries before an evening out. Avoid showers that are too hot, which can cause problems falling asleep.

POST-SPORT COMFORT

It eliminates knots in the muscles and the sweat of exercise, chlorine from the swimming pool ...

HYDROTHERAPY AT HOME

Multiple water jets, massages, steam cabins—there's no limit to the manufacturers' imaginations. And the bathroom is increasingly becoming a living space all on its own.

60 litres for a shower compared to 150 litres for a (deep) bath
Ecology seems to have chosen sides ... unless you spend 20 minutes under the shower.

A 'Scottish shower',
which has come to mean 'running hot and cold' in a figurative sense, is derived from actual hydrotherapy practices in 19th-century Scotland.

THE WORD FROM THE DERMATOLOGIST
Showers clean the skin, but also dry it out. Body oils and nourishing shower gels are a must ... before moving on to the moisturising phase!

Years, fatigue…
scrub it all away!

Exfoliating to make new skin is 'the' survival reflex for our little cells … Here again, it's most important not to leave the body behind!

THE WORD FROM THE DERMATOLOGIST WELCOME TO SCRUBBING!

A scrub, or exfoliation cream, is an extremely effective partnership between little abrasive granules coated in a cream that provides all the necessary gentleness. There are hordes of special body formulas offering specific benefits according to their active ingredients.

THE PLUSES

Not only does it **refine the texture** of the skin, but the practice of exfoliation also lays down a red carpet for the active ingredients in other products that are applied (slimming, relaxing, nourishing, moisturising) and makes them **more effective** on skin that's more permeable.

ATTACK FROM ABOVE

A generous dose of exfoliating scrub for the **shoulders** and **arms**, using circular movements to rub. **Use scrub** on the back of the arms and especially the **elbows**, key zones which easily become rough and take on an unappealing chapped appearance. Go more gently on the décolletage—which should not, however, be neglected—and especially the breasts, to be taken care of in all daily routines.

SATINY LEGS Move up from the **ankles** along the **calves** (perfect before a hair-removal session), paying special attention to the **knees**, then the **thighs** and **buttocks**, still using circular movements for incredible softness.

WHEN?

Ideally, once a week (no more than twice, in any case, at the risk of irritating the epidermis), in the shower, to take advantage of having damp skin … and of being able to rinse off completely, leaving no trace of the little exfoliating granules.

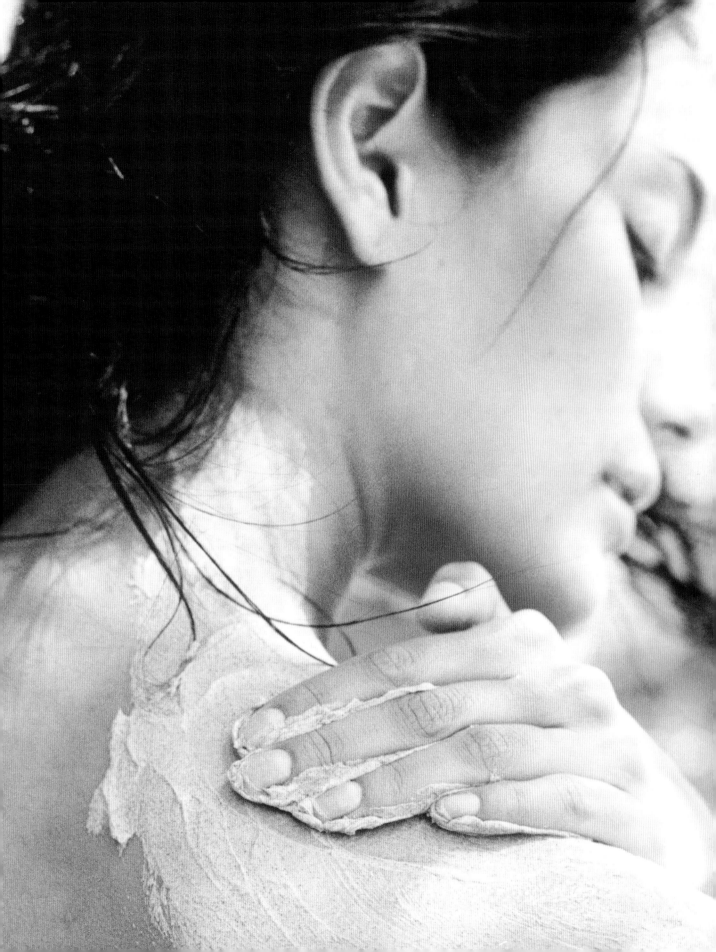

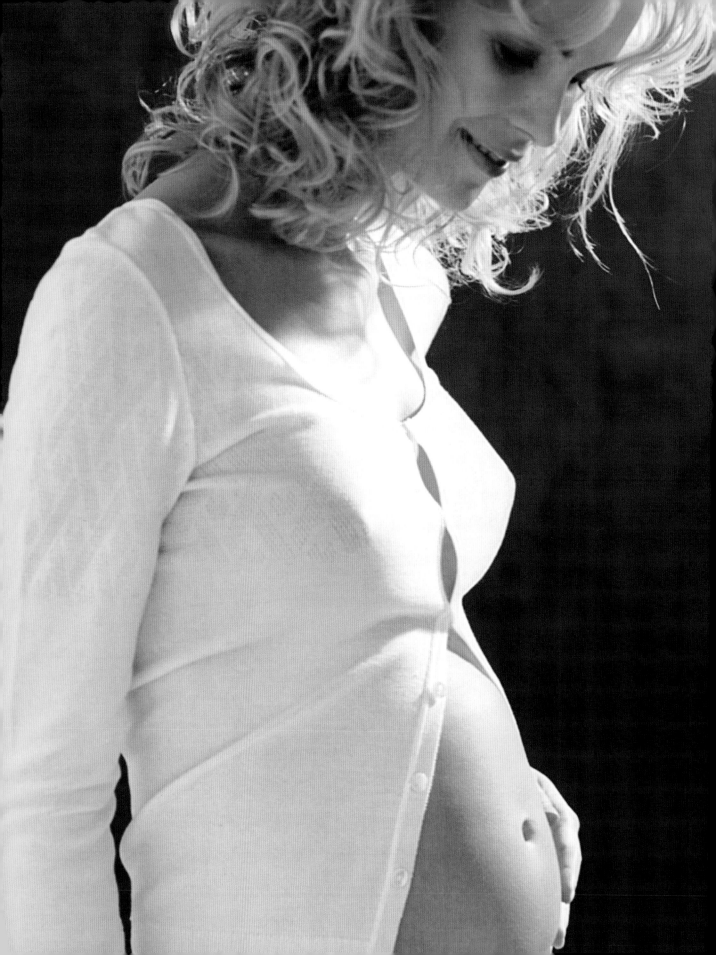

Lovely
future mum

*Pregnancy is an extraordinary physiological interlude,
a serene journey offering supreme fulfilment ... but a time when,
more than ever, we should pamper ourselves.*

WITH 100,000 TIMES MORE HORMONES... your skin is saturated with water, stored up with salt at the level of the dermis. The immediate effect of this ultra-hydration: an incredible radiance. The oestrogens also tidy things up: excess seborrhoea and acne conditions improve greatly in 99% of cases.

PREVENTING STRETCH MARKS Skin fibres, when subjected to too much pressure, can tear in some people at the level of the dermis, where the collagen and elastin are found. The only solution is to constantly moisturise the stomach, breasts, hips and the tops of the thighs, at least every morning and evening. Ultra-nourishing, special stretch-mark formulas will capture the moisture molecules.

THE MASK UNDERNEATH Since the synthesis of melanin is itself boosted, use total sunblock without exception.

WEIGHT GAIN should be limited and monitored. Even if most of the problems can be rectified afterwards, it's better if the skin hasn't been overstretched. Superficial cellulite is another result of the significant rise in hormone levels. Drink lots of water, have a low-salt diet and a few draining massages.

STAY FIRM... BUT GENTLE

A short list of recommended activities (bra essential!): **walking, swimming, gentle exercises, yoga, stretching, water exercises, (indoor!) cycling**.

T minus one week
- hair removal + haircut
- manicure + pedicure.

To slip into the maternity beauty kit
- dry shampoo
- moisturising towellettes
- mild fragrance-free deodorant
- mineral water mister
- bronzing powder for dull skin
- mascara ... a waterproof one!

THE WORD FROM THE ANGIOLOGIST
- Be vigilant: 20% of varicose veins appear during the first pregnancy, 40% during the second...
- Being more or less vulnerable to getting stretch marks is hereditary. Your mum had them? Never mind! Your genetic heritage might come from your father!
- Our 'fat reserves' build up to enable us to breastfeed.

Hydration
at the source

A daily expectation of the body as well as the face: restoring the skin's moisture balance is a priority for personal health.

IT'S FOR OUR OWN PROTECTION

… that our skin is impermeable to water! Otherwise, we couldn't take a bath without turning into a giant sponge. But the water we drink daily (and which is in our food) constantly escapes from us (as perspiration), hence the necessity of inventing ways to preserve it naturally by strengthening our passive defence mechanisms.

HELP, I'VE BEEN FORGOTTEN!

Apart from in summer (when the beach demands it), we are much too inclined to overlook moisturising our body, which is nevertheless the front line of defence against threats (water at the top of the list, but also temperature variations, excess sun exposure, stress …).

COLD DEHYDRATES... as much as heat!

The skin on the legs and arms, which is particularly low in sebaceous glands, suffers in winter. We protect our body with warm clothes … but we must also provide our skin with an appropriate cosmetic 'wardrobe'.

Daily use of a nourishing and moisturising treatment helps the skin to reinforce its natural protection. This protective microlayer acts in a way comparable to sebum, the basis of the fine hydrolipidic film our skin can't do without.

Water tricks
If you are plunged into water up to your neck, even if you are completely dehydrated, you lose all sensation of thirst!

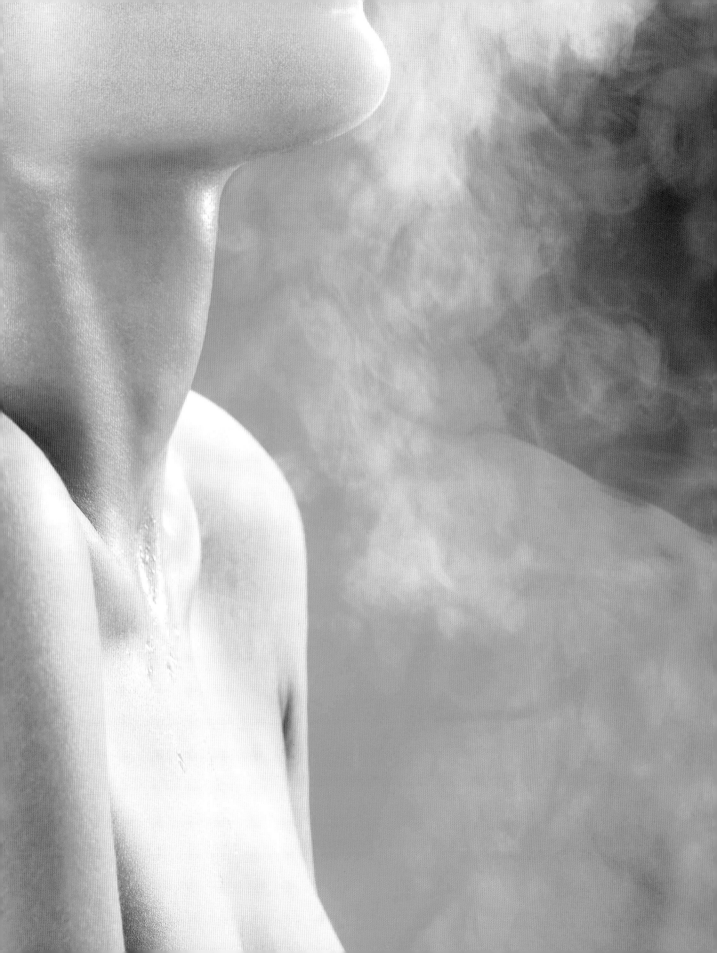

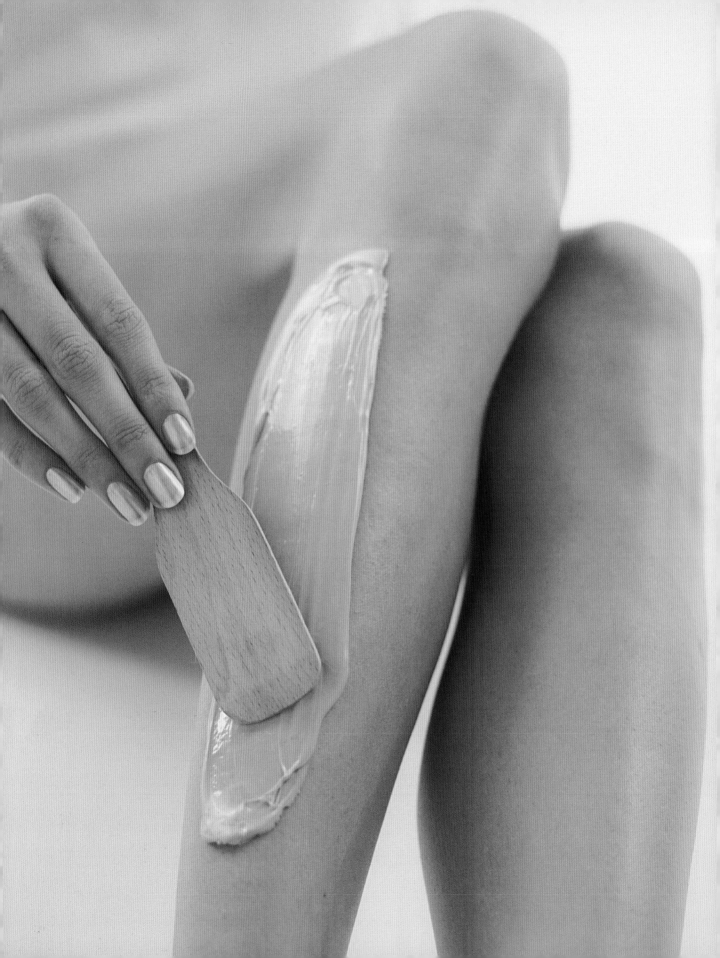

Smooth, hairless: razing the myths

Satiny legs, bikini line and armpits that I prefer ... clean. Solutions that hit the spot for smooth skin.

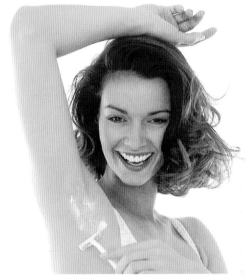

WAX It gets the prize for efficiency and longevity, and there are now more flexible textures. At home for experts or preferably at the beautician's, for more dexterity (and the back of the legs!). Two musts: a disposable one-use wax (for hygiene) applied lukewarm (to avoid problems with veins). Talcum powder between each strip protects from irritations.

To limit ingrown hairs: exfoliation before waxing (never with a horsehair glove) and repeated moisturising afterwards, with special anti-regrowth formulas. And **tweezers** for touch-ups. A traditional Middle Eastern variation: a delicious mixture of sugar and honey.

SHAVING For emergencies, it remains an entirely valid option. But even if it doesn't stimulate regrowth, the fact that it cuts the hair at skin level means the remaining hair is thicker ... and it prickles! For comfort levels, there are inbuilt skin conditioners or foams, and take advantage of the bath for better-prepared skin.

DEPILATORY CREAMS To be handled with care, and after testing beforehand (patch test 24 hours before). Rinse off under the shower, but avoid using soap to prevent irritations.

ELECTRIC DEPILATOR A very attractive alternative to shaving, to the extent that it tears out (part of) the roots. It is also much kinder, with anaesthetising versions (using cold gel). The effect can be reproduced by rubbing an ice cube over beforehand!

BLEACHING Preferable for the face and arms, except in extreme cases.

The right age to start? As late as possible, to avoid turning adolescent downiness into real fur.

THE WORD FROM THE COSMETIC DOCTOR

For long-term hair removal (the word 'permanent' is no longer used), intense pulsed light (IPL) is used to penetrate the melanin of the hair and destroy the root. More effective and less painful than previous methods (including lasers) on pigmented hair, it remains a long-term process, over several months, with yearly follow-up sessions.

Which formula
for whom?

How do you find your way through the profusion of pots and bottles? A brief guide to the different textures, so you can get the best out of them!

THE WORD FROM THE PHARMACIST BRIGITTE LEROUX (Lierac)

It's best not to be too quick to judge a product: it takes 21 to 40 days to assess the effectiveness of a treatment—the time it takes the cells to renew themselves. Disappointment is sometimes the result of not using a product properly! The multiplicity of differently textured products isn't a marketing ploy: the different formulations are not interchangeable. When it comes to sunscreens, for example, a cream will be more effective than a spray with the same protection factor.

MASKS

With longer application times and extra-powerful ingredients, they manage systematic problems over time or as stand-alone therapy.

SERUMS

With a high concentration of active ingredients and quick absorption, they complement or boost the action of the treatment applied on top of them. To be used throughout the year or as a special treatment, when the skin is tired.

CREAMS

A superlative texture, the queen of moisturising and anti-age treatments … usually rich and smooth.

MILKS

More liquid than creams, they quickly penetrate the skin. Ideal for the body: you can get dressed straightaway after application.

FLUIDS

Also called emulsions. Fine and light, fluids are designed for combination-style skins or warm climates.

GELS

Most often transparent, they don't leave any greasy film on the skin and guarantee a feeling of freshness.

OILS

Ideal for giving the body a satiny finish (very sexy glossy effect). Dry oils penetrate the skin very quickly without any greasy residue.

SPRAYS

Light and fresh, perfect for sunscreens that are applied repeatedly and for difficult-to-reach areas like the back.

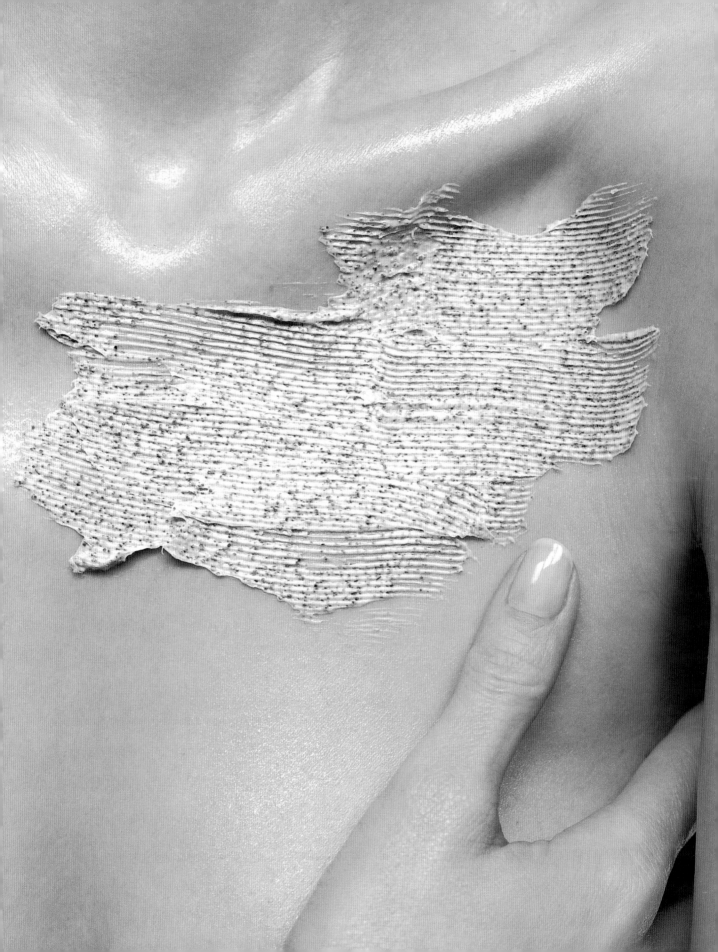

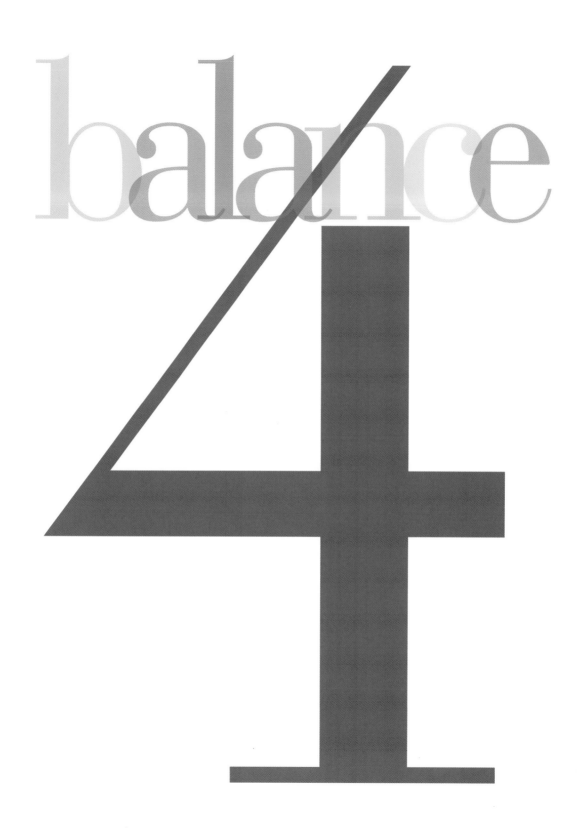

balance

4

MY FIGURE

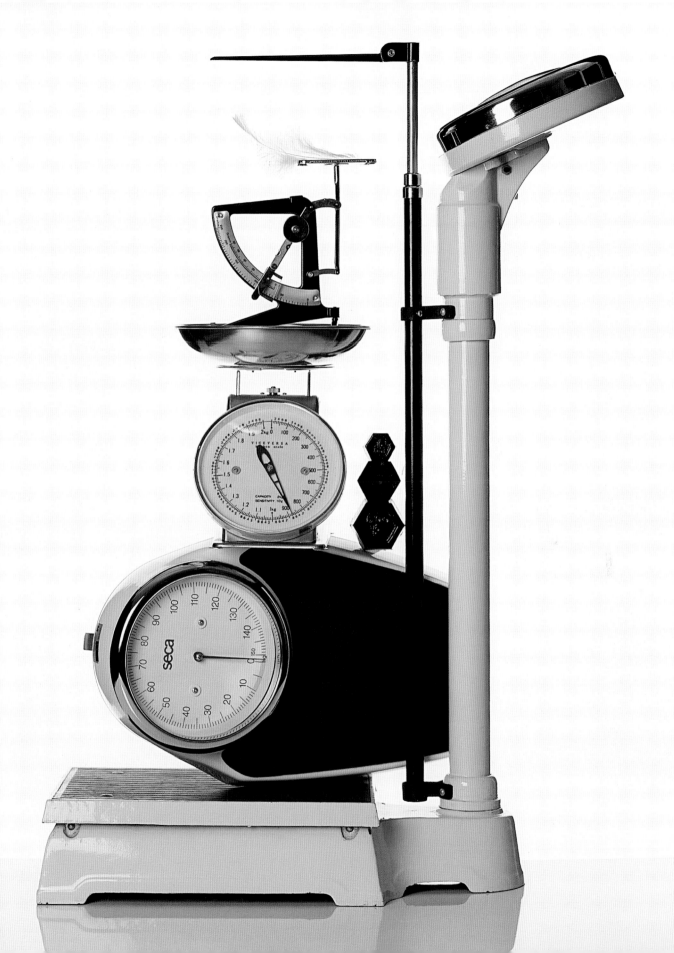

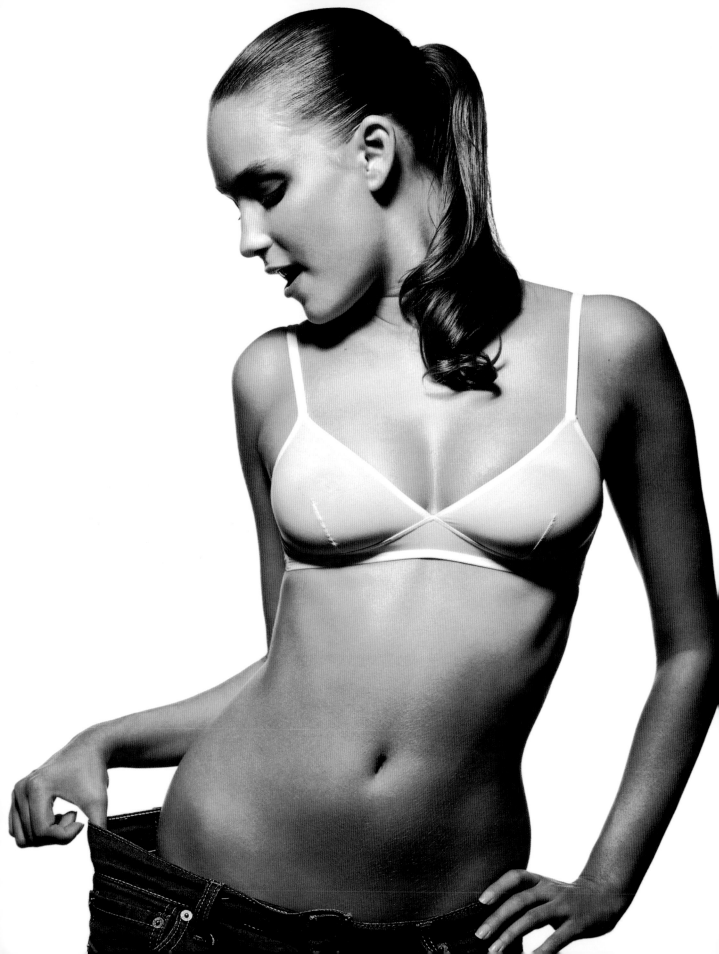

Streamlining your goals

Firm
in your aims

Trying to get rid of our No 1 hereditary enemy, cellulite?
Fine, but don't lose your head or your femininity: jettisoning
uncomfortable and inelegant extra bulges has nothing to do
with obsessively tracking that unfortunate extra gram.

GRACEFUL SHAPES

Our **body's fat deposits** are governed by hormones, like our veins. The fat cells in the vulnerable zones will fill out below the belt (this is the 'gynoid' body type, whereas men get … a bellyful!) before spreading to the rest of the body. Practically no woman is spared from this process—even the thinnest ones have their dimples.

Depending on the metabolism, this fatty mass represents **10 to 25% of our weight**. It is made up of cells with high lipid levels, the adipocytes (fat cells), grouped into fatty deposits that are imprisoned in a network of walls of connective tissue and criss-crossed by lymph and blood vessels and nerve fibres. It contains 10 to 15% water.

Adipocytes are extendable cells that can store a significant amount of fat as they **can increase in volume up to 27 times**. Fats are stored in the adipocytes in the form of **triglycerides**, molecules synthesised inside the adipocyte using glucose and free fatty acids. This is the principle of lipogenesis (the production of fat); at the other end of the spectrum **lipolysis** performs the breakdown of fats. But, under the influence of various factors (hormones, dietary intake above the body's energy needs), there is an increase in **lipogenesis**. An imbalance develops between storage and use—this is the origin of the formation and depositing of cellulite. ▶

Extra belly padding?
You just have to pinch the skin between two fingers while pushing down to the muscle belt, measure and divide by two to get the thickness of the fat layer. Above 1.5 cm, the answer is yes!

THE WORD FROM THE DOCTOR, DR CLAUDE GARDE
There are numerous definitions of cellulite put foward by medical histologists (tissue specialists). The most precise one is 'hydrolipodystrophy', which suggests both the accumulation of fat cells and the bulging due to the water trapped inside the tissues.

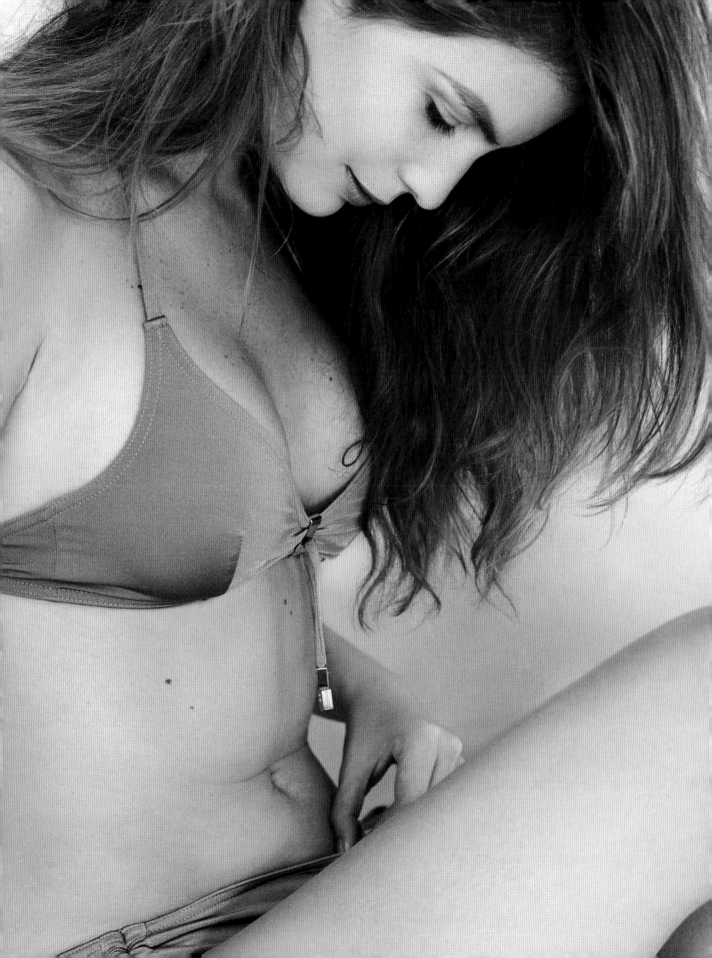

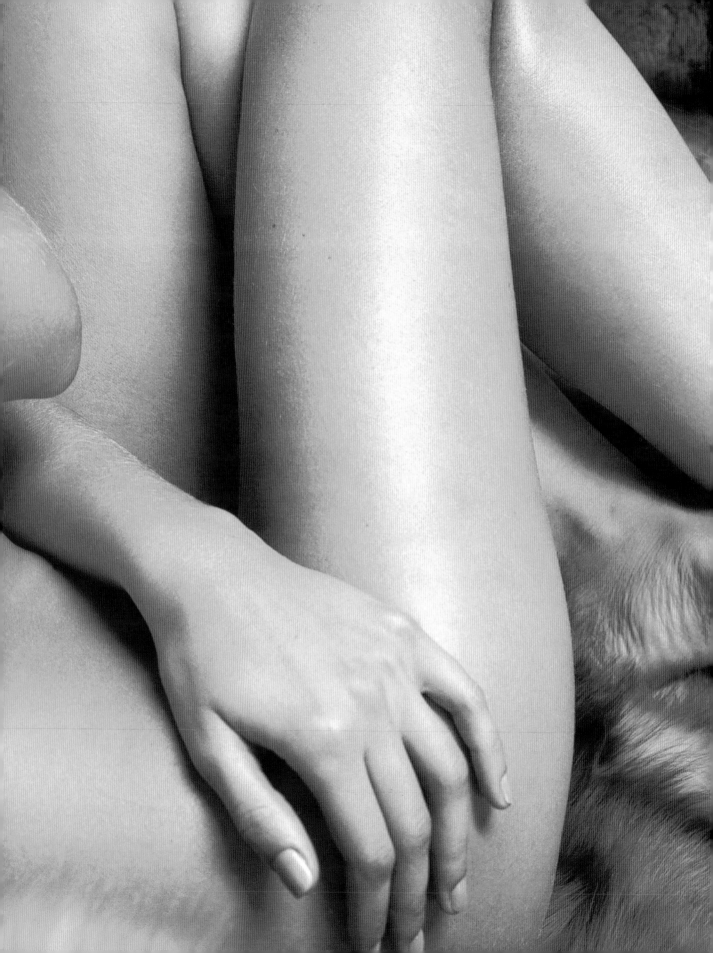

▶ CELLULITE UNDER THE MICROSCOPE

Cellulite affects all women, to a greater or lesser extent: the least hormonal imbalance can serve as a trigger.

It's often the first contraceptive pill that sets off or increases deposits of cellulite. Pregnancy tends to encourage the development of heavier thighs or 'saddlebags'. The adipocytes are endowed with regulating receptors, which encourage the synthesis of fat on the thighs and buttocks. The different distribution of fat at menopause, on the hips and abdomen, is connected to a lower production of feminine hormones.

Surface cellulite develops in accordance with the same rhythm, often stimulated by hormone-based contraceptives, then hormone replacements. But it is more sensitive to variations in the amount of water in the tissues, which explains why the appearance of cellulite fluctuates a great deal, sometimes even according to the phase of the menstrual cycle.

Aggravating factors are age, which gradually slows down the metabolism, and also hereditary or ethnic factors (the generosity of Mediterranean curves is not a myth).

THE BMI: ALWAYS A GOOD GUIDE?

The **BMI (body mass index)** = weight divided by height squared (it can be easily calculated for you on the Internet):

- less than 24.9: normal (less than 18.5: anorexia alert!)
- between 25 and 29.9: overweight
- over 30: obesity.

A young woman 1.65 m tall can weigh an average of 50 to 65 kg. She will be considered obese above 80 kg. **Warning: these parameters vary according to age and body type**.

We are far from the beauty ideals of centuries past, when a large-bottomed figure was a sign of good health. Equality isn't what it used to be in the kingdom of thin legs and short skirts. At the same time, medicine has discovered another vocation for itself in the service of beauty ... as long as beauty and health follow the same path. The resolution of apparently aesthetic problems improves the prognosis for our life and vital functions: living better, longer and more beautiful.

THE WORD FROM THE COACH Scales offering biometrical impedance analysis (BIA) allow body fat to be measured (as well as other valuable biological information) instead of just being restricted to measuring weight.

Taking myself in hand

When you grasp the problem with both hands you get results.
As long as you keep it up: daily attention is essential.
The key? Targeted massages for smooth, toned skin, and a genuine
impact on cellulite (and spider veins)!

Turn down the heat
The body uses more energy if it has to ward off the cold. **Water represents** only 30% of the weight of the adipose (fatty) tissue: losing weight is hard work. Hence the need to drink more water to facilitate the work of the kidneys in eliminating impurities.

THE WORD FROM THE DOCTOR
'ORANGE PEEL SKIN'
Also called surface cellulite, as opposed to deep-level cellulite or fatty deposits. It represents a genuine 'padding' that covers the lower limbs fairly evenly and also the upper body. It is packed with water and finds itself trapped in little pockets of fibrous tissue, which prevents the microcirculation from doing its job perfectly. It is very sensitive to female hormones and especially progesterone. This is what gives the skin its dimpled appearance.

BREAK DOWN THE LUMPS!
For a minimum of 4 weeks, every day after showering, apply a slimming cream or gel rich in active ingredients that drain and break down fats, retained water and toxins (caffeine, bitter orange, ivy, horse chestnut, ginkgo biloba, calcium, soy extract), **boosted by massage.**

The right start: dietary supplements that combat fat and water retention (blackcurrant, green tea, dandelion).

CLASSIC MASSAGE
Using **circular movements**, move from the ankles to the tops of the thighs, finishing with the hips and buttocks.

ULTRA-PROFESSIONAL: MANUAL VENOUS DRAINAGE
More effectively eliminates the water trapped in the vein tissue by allowing the bloodflow to return to a more logical course. The deep vein network (inside the muscles) and the surface network (between the muscles and the skin) communicate via (perforating) 'siphons', which are stimulated by this technique.

Sit with your legs stretched out, bend the leg to be massaged. Start with the inside of the foot, then move up towards the groin via the inside leg and thigh. Repeat 10 times, stretching out the leg again when you reach the groin. **For the front of the thigh**, move from the outside of the knee up to the groin. **For the outside thigh**, start from the top of the thigh, moving down towards the back of the knee. **For the lower leg—calf, knee and ankle—**always work from bottom to top and **for the hips**, from the outside inwards towards the groin. Finish with the **feet on the wall**, lying on the back, making windscreen-wiper movements.

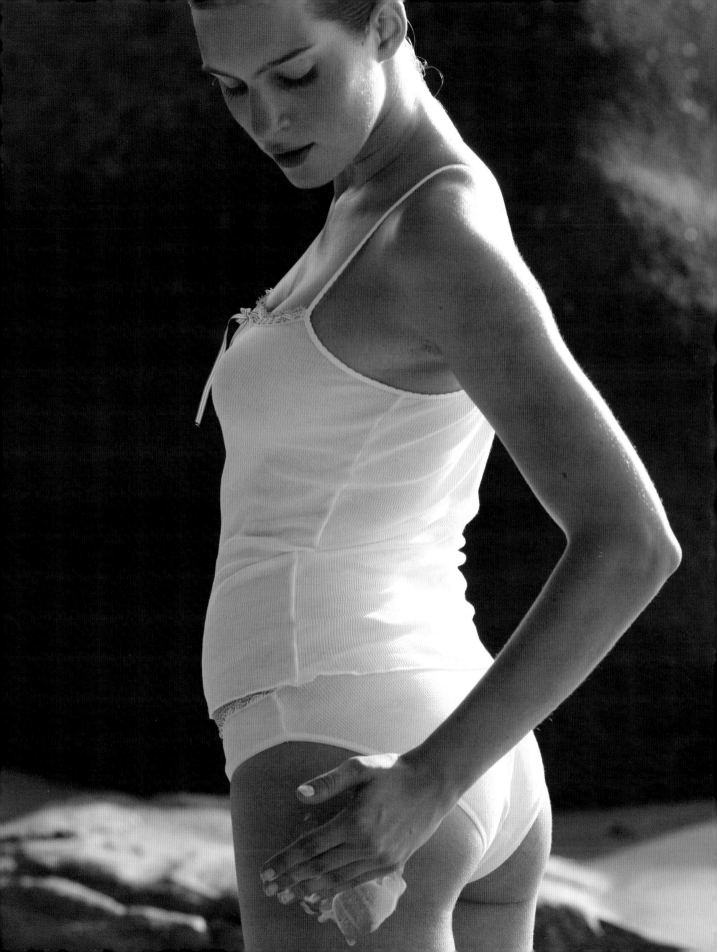

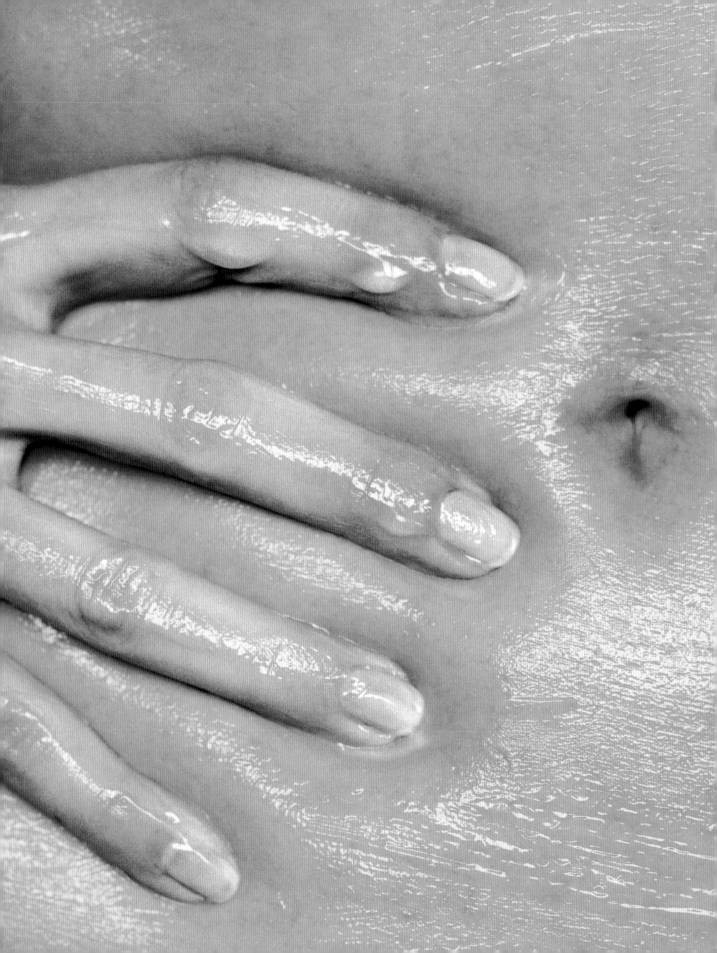

Liposuction
cases in point

Proven techniques, an unquestionably aesthetic but rigorously medical approach: a brief annotated guide to the options.

The starting point is to eliminate any potentially aggravating factors (problems with the **hormones, circulation**…).

Injections, ultrasounds, pinch-and-roll massage, lymphatic drainage—apart from sport and exercise, the range of treatments that break down cellulite are covered. **Mesotherapy** (the injection of products using a very short needle) is effective for localised cellulite deposits.

THE STOMACH is a favourite site for small fat deposits, as well as for all the tensions (and distensions): at the top of the list, pregnancy, which sometimes distends the skin and the muscle belt. What to do? If it's just a little paunch, a **liposuction** procedure under local anaesthetic will effectively resolve the problem, but surgery may understandably seem dramatic and to be reserved rather for larger volumes. A **hydrotomy** (or **lipoclasis** or **lipolysis**) procedure offers the same result without any surgical incision, hospitalisation or the need for follow-up treatment. The effectiveness of **lipolaser** or **laser lipolysis procedures** is now universally recognised as an outpatient procedure, without follow-up treatments or the need to take time off work.

When there are several problems occurring together (distended muscle and skin, significant fat thickness), an **abdominoplasty** ('tummy tuck') is necessary. A serious operation, not without its risks, which leaves a significant scar. Think carefully before undertaking one!

THE WORD FROM THE SURGEON
WHEN THE MUSCULAR ENVELOPE HAS BECOME SLACK: this is expressed on the abdominal level by a widening of the connection between the left and right sides of the main abdominal muscle (diastasis recti or 'abdominal separation'), which pushes the stomach forward even though there is hardly any fat to lose or remove. The solution consists in tightening this central abdominal zone via an incision that will be hidden under a bathing suit.
WHEN THE FAT IS ON THE INSIDE OF THE ABDOMEN (a protruding abdomen, more than 80 cm in circumference), it is a case of a metabolic syndrome, generally associated with excessively high levels of sugar and fat in the blood and hypertension.
▶ This is a medical problem.

MY FIGURE

▶ A TEXTBOOK CASE: THE BUTTOCKS

Losing weight means emptying the container holding the extra kilos: watch out for **ptosis** (drooping) of the buttocks, which, paradoxically, can make the area look heavier. Operating on this area is rather like sculpture: it can be worked on using a table angled at 35/45° to take the effect of gravity into account, with the involvement of the patient (clenching the buttock muscles) and an assortment of different techniques: **lipolysis** or **lipolaser** if it is a case of reducing size, **lipofilling** if it is a case of filling out an area, **lipolaser** to retighten an area, or **liposuction** under general anaesthetic … after carefully weighing up the benefits and risks.

OPERATION LEGS: LIPO WITHOUT STRESS

Progressive ambulatory liposculpture combines the effectiveness of liposuction (eliminating fat through aspiration) with the reduced stress of a procedure carried out under local anaesthetic without the need to take time off work, but in a surgical environment.
Lipolaser for deep cellulite deposits: a less complex procedure than liposuction, it is growing in popularity. **Lipolysis** may be a suggestion for smaller cellulite deposits (hip, knees), and is a very attractive option for surface cellulite or 'orange peel skin' (no aspiration is involved), combined with vacuum therapy to smooth out the surface.

Classic liposuction is not a method of losing weight but of reducing the size of abnormally developed areas. Liposculpture is carried out using a cannula connected to a source of aspiration. At the end of the session (two and a half hours maximum), adhesive bandages or a panty girdle are worn for at least three weeks. The inside of the thighs is the most difficult area to treat: the delicacy of the skin demands a great deal of attention.

The buttocks
Buttocks must always be shown off. They're the most complex, but also the most exciting area for the doctor. The whole difficulty of treating them comes from the fact that they are 'suspended' on a fixed framework and subject to gravity (all buttocks are beautiful lying down on the beach).

A knee pocket?
A formidable fat-storage zone ruled by hormones; an inflammation can encourage the transformation of certain cells into fat cells, by stimulating the process of lipogenesis (the swelling of these reservoirs by the production of fat).

THE WORD FROM THE DOCTOR
Before undertaking any procedure, discuss it in depth with your doctor, as for any non-trivial procedure that uses an anaesthetic.

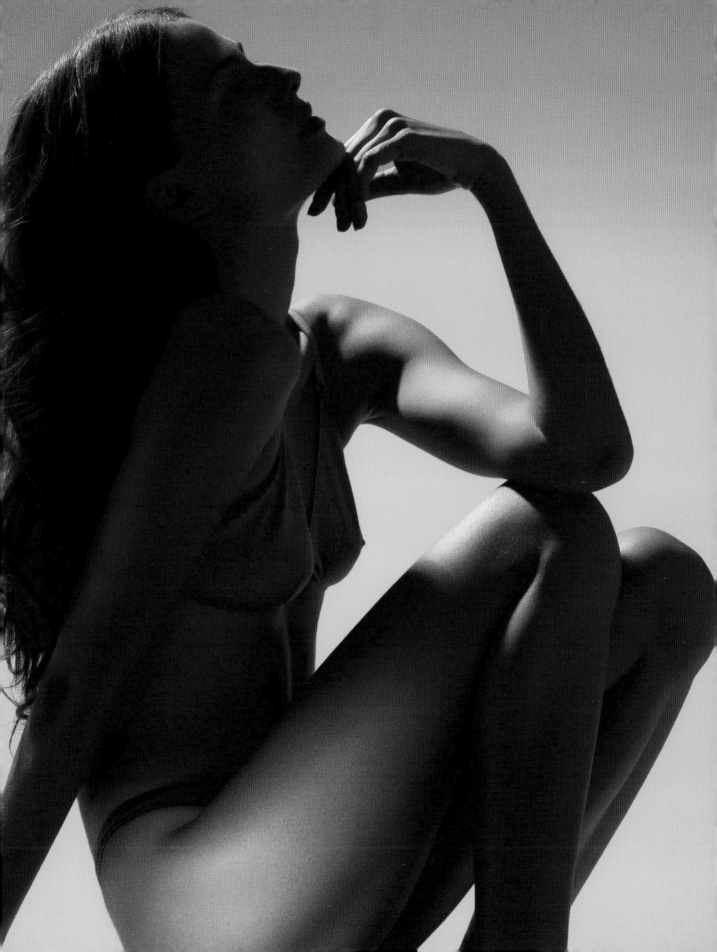

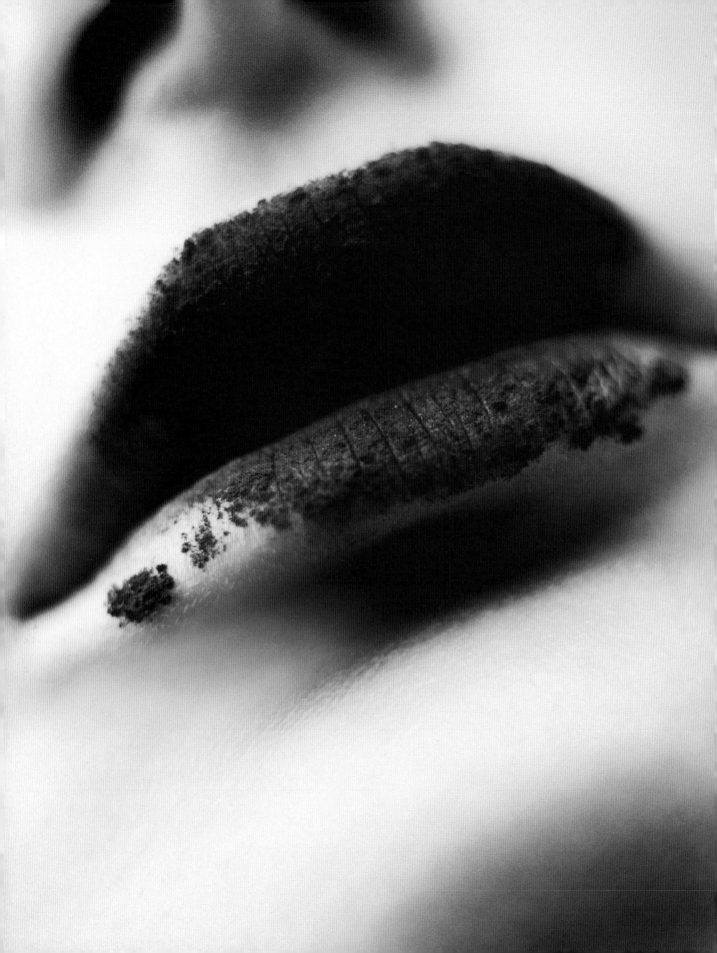

Sink your teeth into life

feast on pleasure

Health
on the table!

It's the foundation of everything else: a balanced diet gets the body running beautifully.

Losing weight from where I want?
This is the goal of morphonutrition:
• too much sugar and vegetables will put weight on the breasts and thighs
• too much carbohydrate will put weight on the stomach
• too much protein will develop the chest and muscles.

Slimming? About time!
The principle behind chrononutrition: finding a dietary rhythm that's a function of your needs. Some 'good' fats in the morning, accompanied by some energy-packed protein to give the body a good start, an energy-rich midday meal, light in the afternoon. And the evening meal: ultra-light!

THE WORD FROM THE DIETITIAN
THE SPICE QUEENS
Cinnamon helps to lower the sugar levels in the blood. Ginger heats the senses with more than 40 antioxidant compounds. It facilitates the digestion of garlic and onion, cooked in the same dish to optimise the effect of the beneficial molecules. And turmeric (see page 117).

IT'S NOT ABOUT DEPRIVING YOURSELF ANY MORE

We've had our fill of crash and fad diets. The sole priority today is choosing the best nourishment for our (beautiful) machine, which will yield nothing but benefits for its motor: the brain. A healthy mind in a healthy body … go further and for longer. The key idea is to **eat less but better**: foods rich in protective ingredients (fibre, antioxidants, magnesium, vitamins and minerals, phyto-oestrogens, with good omega-3 fats). Taking care of the intestine (a 'second brain' and first warning system) means being able to absorb and profit from all of these treats.

PRO PROBIOTICS?

Probiotics are 'live micro-organisms which when administered in adequate amounts confer a health benefit on the host' … Which is to say—us!

The intestine performs the essential functions of digestion, absorption, defence and tolerance. An imbalance in the bacterial flora (stress, poorly tolerated foods, medications …) causes immediate discomfort and leads to health risks in the longer term. Probiotics restore the flora, improve problems with intestinal functions and enable nutrients to be better absorbed.

TELL ME WHAT YOU EAT...

Our **body type** is in part due to our diet.

All of this is mitigated by the role of hormonal receptors located in the fat cells, heredity, ethnicity …

▶

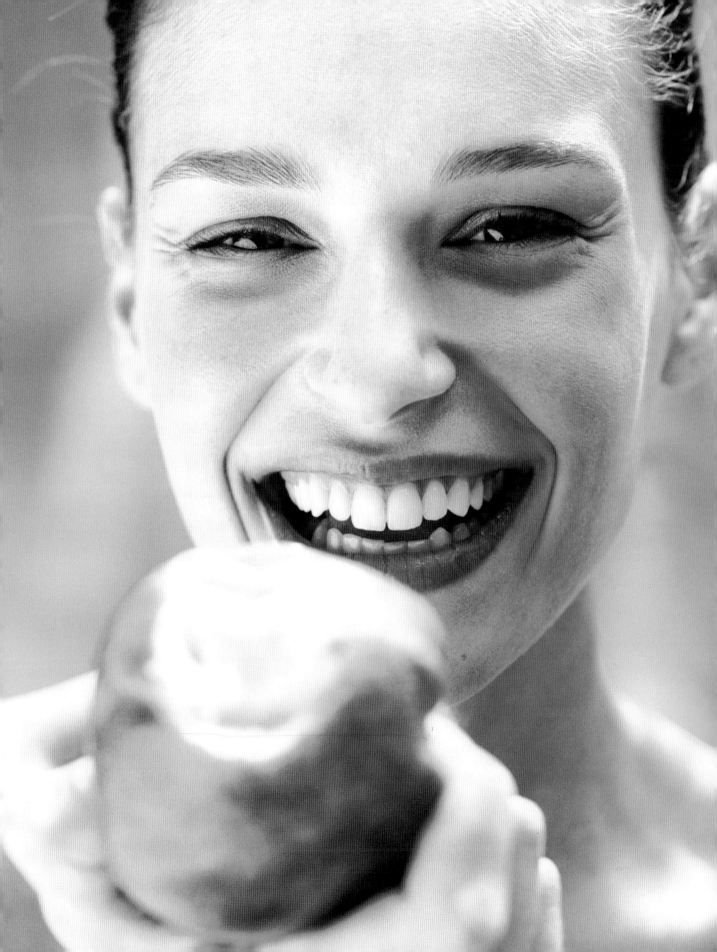

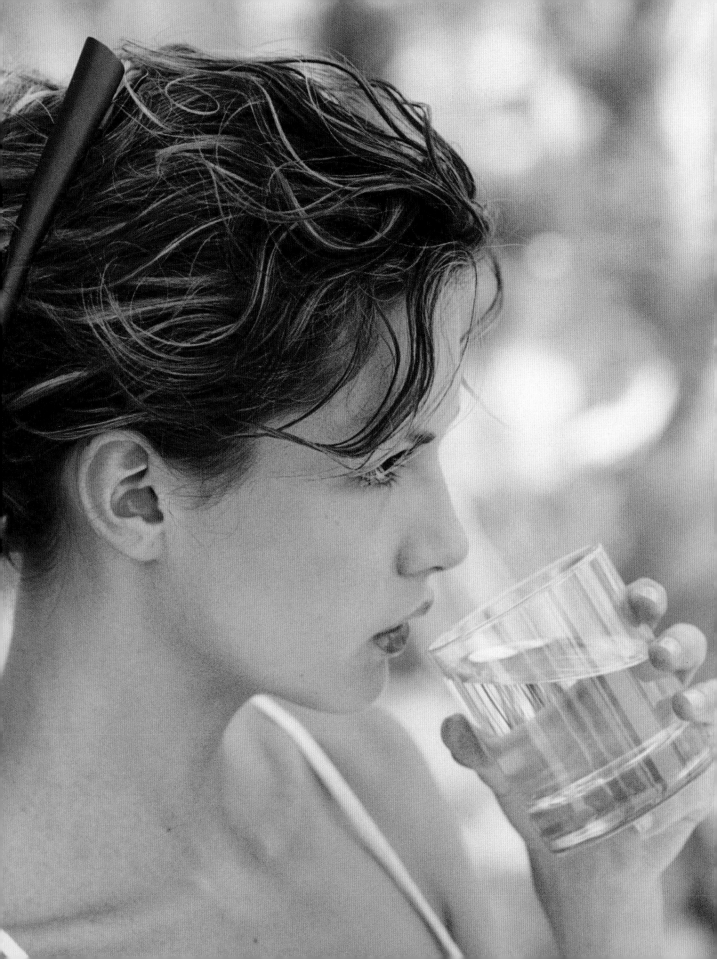

▶ OKINAWA: LONGEVITY ON THE MENU...

All of the **benefits of Japanese cuisine, but even better** (more variety and less salt). The diet and lifestyle of the inhabitants of this archipelago, located on the spice route off the coast of Japan, have been studied for over thirty years. Known for their longevity and proverbial good health, Okinawans don't eat very much, but lots of vegetables, oily fish, soy-based products, seaweed, wholegrain rice, sweet potatoes, dried beans, little meat, no dairy products or wheat (thus no gluten), no sugar, little salt. Finally, they manage stress very well (see Tai chi, page 162) ...

The spice cousin of ginger, turmeric, is unknown in Japan but is used widely on Okinawa. Turmeric is a 'multi-anti': anti-inflammatory, anti-microbial, anti-viral, anti-infectious, anti-tumoral, anti-parasitic.

Cretan-style diets, which are quite similar, add red wine (in moderation, for the benefits of the **resveratrol**) and olive oil (with its **flavonoid**-type antioxidants).

THE ABC OF OMEGAS

Over 60% of our brain is made up of lipids, over 70% of which are omega 3, since the fats are formed from different fatty acids. A good balance between them is essential to keep yourself in good health. The right proportions: a minumum of saturated fats ... and **5 times more omega 6 than omega 3**.

Saturated fatty acids: fatty meat, charcuterie products (delicatessen meats), pastries and baked goods, cheeses.

Monounsaturated fatty acids: olive oil.

Omega 3 polyunsaturated fatty acids: canola oil, oily fish.

Omega 6 polyunsaturated fatty acids: sunflower oil (but omega 6 fatty acids occur in high quantities in commercially produced foods, margarines, biscuits).

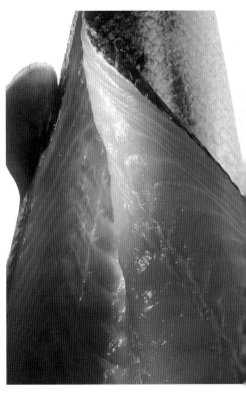

THE WORD FROM THE DIETITIAN
RESOURCES FROM THE SOURCE
1.5 litres of water high in calcium and magnesium.
• Depriving yourself of carbohydrates is a real mistake. Complex carbohydrates are essential carriers of energy, and simply need to be consumed in a measured fashion.

FEAST ON PLEASURE

Fibre, vitamins
and anti-ageing treats

Building up good habits is as good for the morale as for the skin's glow, the beauty of one's hair and nails ... and for balancing your figure.

THE WORD FROM DIETITIAN PATRICIA DUROU

Untoasted, unsalted nuts (walnuts, hazelnuts, almonds, cashew nuts, macadamia nuts, pistachio nuts) are high in good fats, calcium and magnesium and don't cause weight gain (in moderate quantities): the fibre and mineral salt they contain prevents some of the fats from being absorbed.

What about frozen vegetables?

Unless you do your shopping every day, the loss of vitamins is so rapid—half evaporates in two days!—that it would be a shame to deprive yourself of excellent plain vegetables ... which are only waiting to be unfrozen!

AS EVERYDAY TABLE GUESTS...

• fruits and vegetables: in a variety of soups, in salads, gratins, compotes ...

• a few dressed raw vegetables with essential oils (60% olive oil and 40% canola oil, organic and cold-pressed).

• proteins (meat, fish, eggs) in the morning or at midday. Oily fish two or three times per week.

• nuts and dried fruits—figs, prunes, apricots—will liven up salads.

• green tea, rich in polyphenols.

• a light evening meal, but above all containing some carbohydrates.

• a glass and a half of good red wine per day. Just a little coffee, but good quality (preferably organic: pesticides become concentrated in the cup).

ANTIOXIDANTS: A FESTIVAL OF COLOURS

Reds, yellows and oranges (capsicums, apples, tomatoes, citrus fruits, peaches, carrots) for **carotenoids**, **lycopene** and **lutein**.

Purples and violets (red cabbage, beetroot, figs, prunes, dark grapes, blueberries, blackberries, blackcurrants) for **anthocyanins.**

Greens (lettuces, spinach, cabbage) for **chlorophyll**: the green hides the warmer colours, but they—and their benefits—are still there.

CHOCOLATE: BITTERSWEET PLEASURE?

Some of the substances it contains are said to be addictive ... but we're especially hooked on the pleasure of eating it!

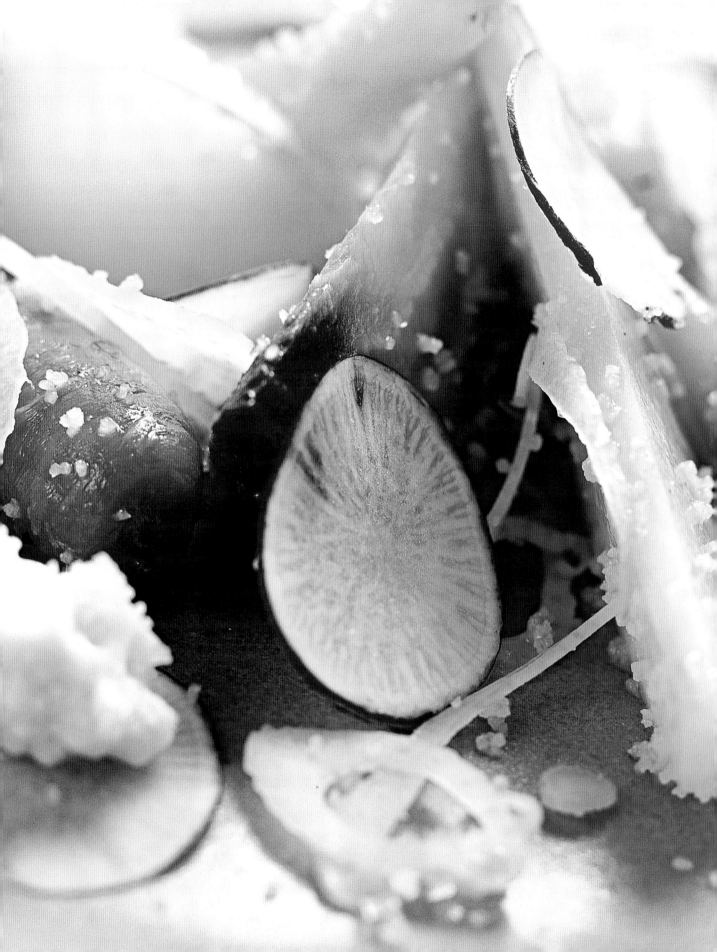

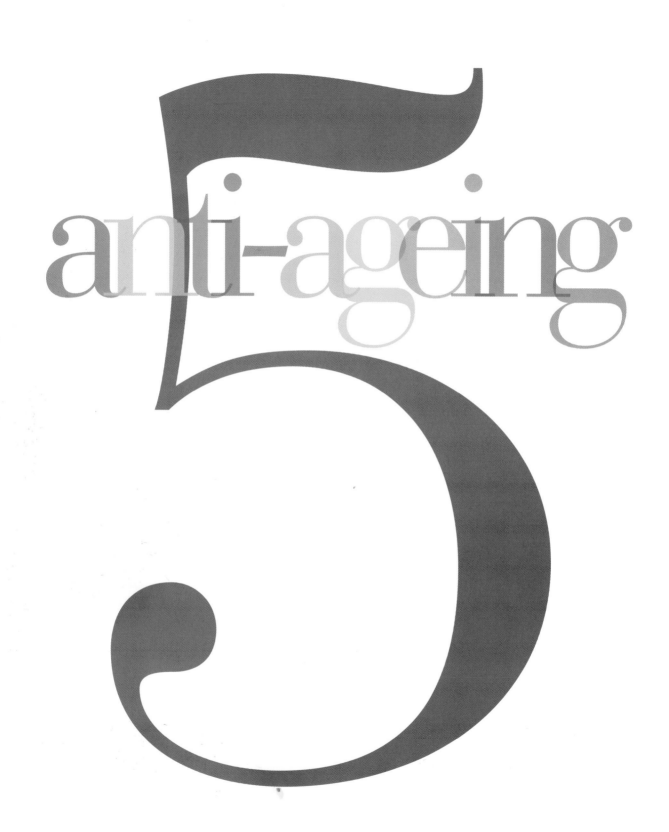

anti-ageing

5

TAMING TIME

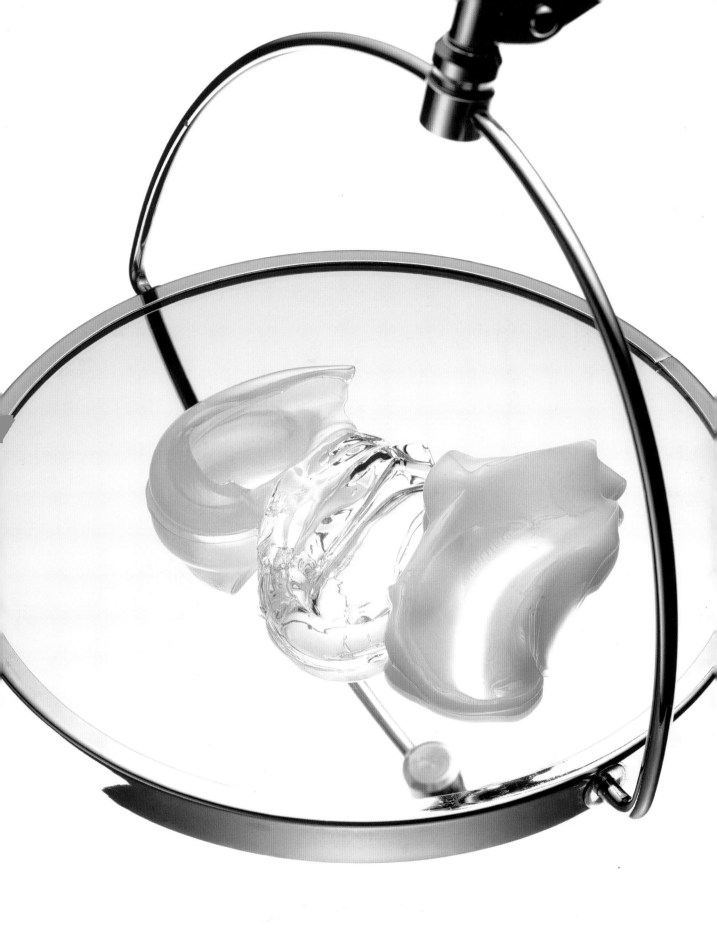

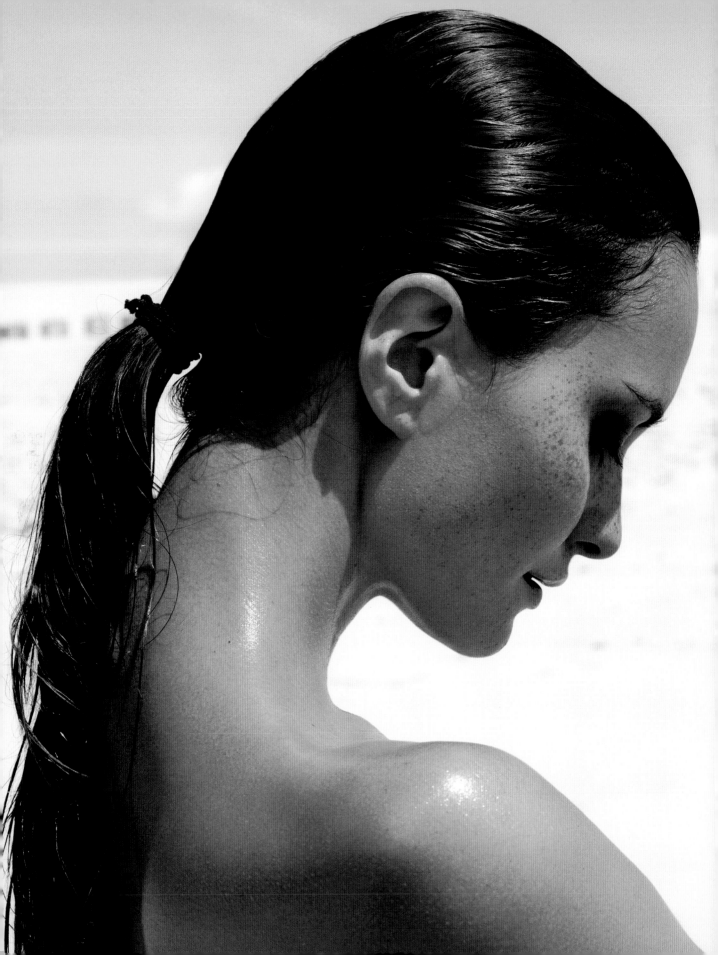

Harnessing and mastering the fullness of time

Doctor, how old is my skin?

A first in this field, the skin biology laboratory directed by Professor Philippe Humbert, head of the dermatology clinic at the Saint-Jacques hospital complex in Besançon, allows us to take a personalised approach to ageing.

A skin and body diagnosis as precise as a medical diagnosis? We are able to calculate the area of the skin's surface and evaluate its 'mechanical' properties (as a function of age and genetic background). Thanks to image-analysis technology, we are able to characterise the type of ageing, identify the therapeutic approach that specifically responds to each case, including the choice of this or that cosmetic product.

Skin elasticity diminishes with age, whereas its **extensibility** increases (by about 5% every 10 years).

- **relief**: this measurement allows the skin's roughness to be assessed, and to count the furrows and plateaux on its surface.
- **complexion and radiance** is measured using an optical device called an eclascope, which studies the skin's light-reflective properties.
- **microcirculation** is quantified by analysis of the skin's small blood vessels, visualised using videocapillaroscopy. A small camera observes the capillary blood vessels through the skin using a process of transillumination (shining light through the skin). **The colour and complexion of the skin** depends in part on these blood vessels' number and distribution.
- **the level of hydration**: an electrical measure, skin capacitance, classifies dry skins according to their 'hydration index' (an HI less than 40 = very dry skin).
- **level of sebum secretion**: a Sebumeter uses a method based on image analysis.

Cosmetic dermatology, recognised by the Société Française de Dermatologie (French Society of Dermatology) and the ISD (International Society of Dermatology), and practised by doctors, has a great deal invested in its rigour and scientific approach. It has many effective modes of treatment at its disposal. It's essential that a precise diagnosis be carried out to define the kind of ageing and also to monitor the effects of the treatments administered. Dermatologists' rooms will gradually become equipped with diagnostic tools based on bio-engineering, biometrology and quantitative imaging.

▶

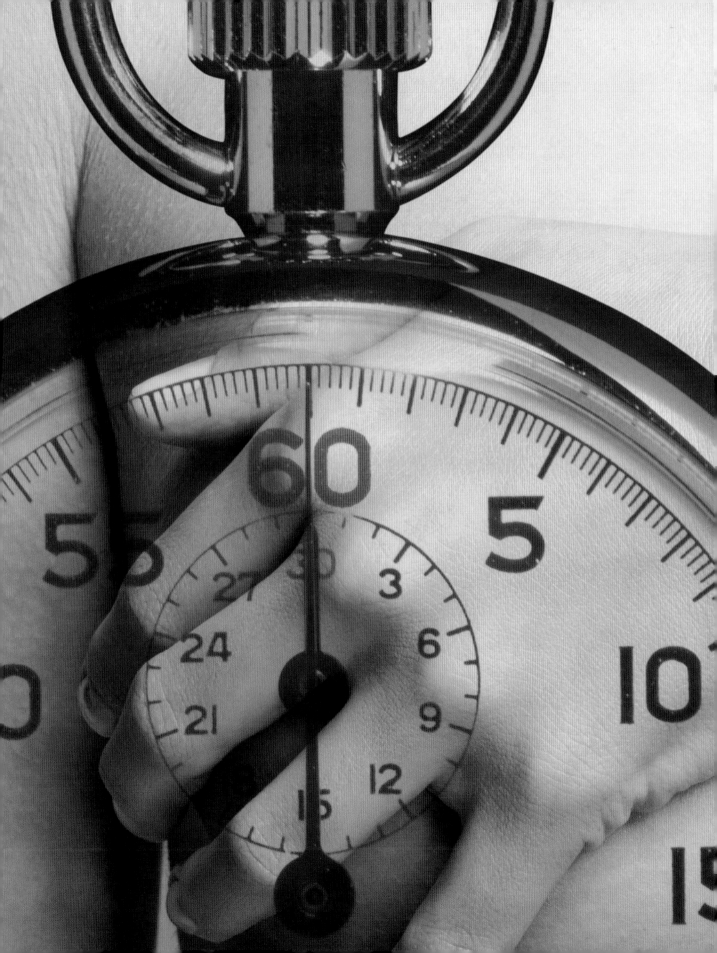

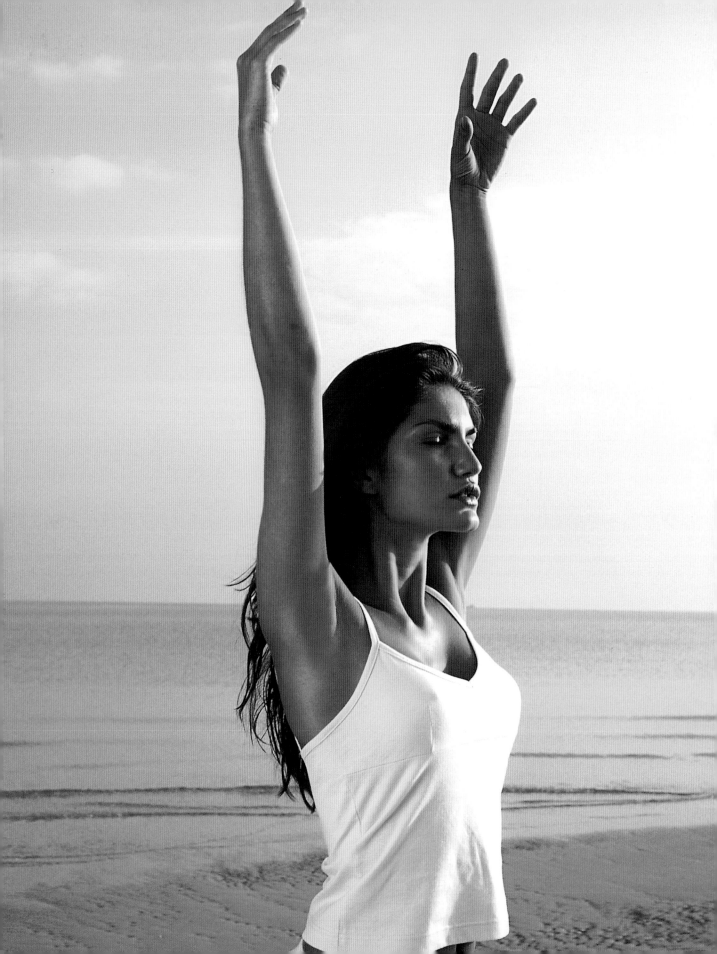

▶ **GOLDEN RULES FOR WARDING OFF THE ENCROACHMENTS OF TIME**

Taking control of the ageing process means, above all, protection and prevention. Sun protection, throwing out the tobacco, eliminating stress … It's taking care of your skin, hydrating it using creams, massaging it using cosmetic products with proven effectiveness.

A holistic approach needs to be taken, to restore the balance (homeostasis) of all of the body's functions—in which nutritional balance plays an integral part.

It's essential to act on every level simultaneously. Otherwise, it's just like reinflating one of four flat tyres!

Cosmetology remains the foundation, acting both on the simple functions such as the skin's protective barrier or the skin's state of hydration. It acts through particular active ingredients, on different cellular functions, allowing cells such as the fibroblasts to be reactivated, or increasing the synthesis of collagen.

Their effectiveness can't be assessed until they have been used for a sufficient length of time, and it's essential to know how to combine active ingredients over time.

There's a noticeable **trend towards using cell therapy as way of controlling the ageing process**. This therapy involves extracting some of a patient's adipose tissue (fatty subcutaneous tissue) and then reinjecting it in certain areas to modify their volume. There's also a trend towards cell therapies using fibroblasts, cells which manufacture collagen within the dermis.

Stem cells, given their multiple potential uses, are especially well-studied in many domains, but also in the area of skin ageing. These methods nevertheless remain difficult to put into practice, costly and still underassessed.

Vitamin C: essential for maintaining the structure of collagen
The reduction in the skin's vitamin C levels as a function of age has been demonstrated in the skin biology laboratory. The measurement curves show, for example, that at 80 years of age the level of vitamin C in the skin has dropped by 50% compared to the skin at 40 years of age.

TAMING TIME

The flower of youth
reaping the fruits

Although we've only been able to extract them since the nineteenth century, the fabulous powers of some plant ingredients have been known since antiquity. Here are some of the fruits of the latest research into nutrition …

THE WORD FROM PROFESSOR MARIE-THÉRÈSE LECCIA
The only molecule whose effectiveness against the skin ageing process has really been demonstrated, by scientific research, on human beings is the acid form of vitamin A (tretinoin). Many cosmetic products, in particular those which claim to have antioxidant properties, have real and very interesting effects in the laboratory, in vitro (the stimulation of collagen, decrease in the breakdown of elastin fibres). But on a living human being, in vivo, it's more difficult to prove. The active ingredients extracted from plants such as green tea are of interest for many reasons, but here again there has not been an evaluation of its effect on the skin ageing process in human beings.

A TOAST TO RESVERATROL!

One of the explanations of the **French paradox** is supposed to be the beneficial role of red wine in moderate doses. It is pointed out that red wine contains high levels of **resveratrol**, a phenolic derivative that occurs in plants, with antioxidant, antiplatelet, anti-inflammatory and vasodilator effects, and preventing the proliferation of cells. It gives cheeks a rosy glow (if consumed in moderation) and extends the life of yeasts by 70%! A University of Quebec researcher, Frédéric Le Cren, flagbearer of the antioxidant revolution, recommends a daily dose, whether taken as a supplement, a bunch of grapes, half a litre of grape juice or … a glass and a half of red wine. Cheers!

GREEN TEA, NOT JUST HYPE

For washing down sushi or a beautiful start to the day, no need to consume in moderation here: green tea combats the troublesome accumulation of fat around the stomach, which is as inelegant as it is potentially harmful (it accelerates ageing and influences diabetes).

POMEGRANATE, AN ANTIOXIDISATION GRENADE

Pomegranate juice, which contains a powerful antioxidant, is supposed to have the potential to inhibit the growth of certain cancers, including breast cancer.

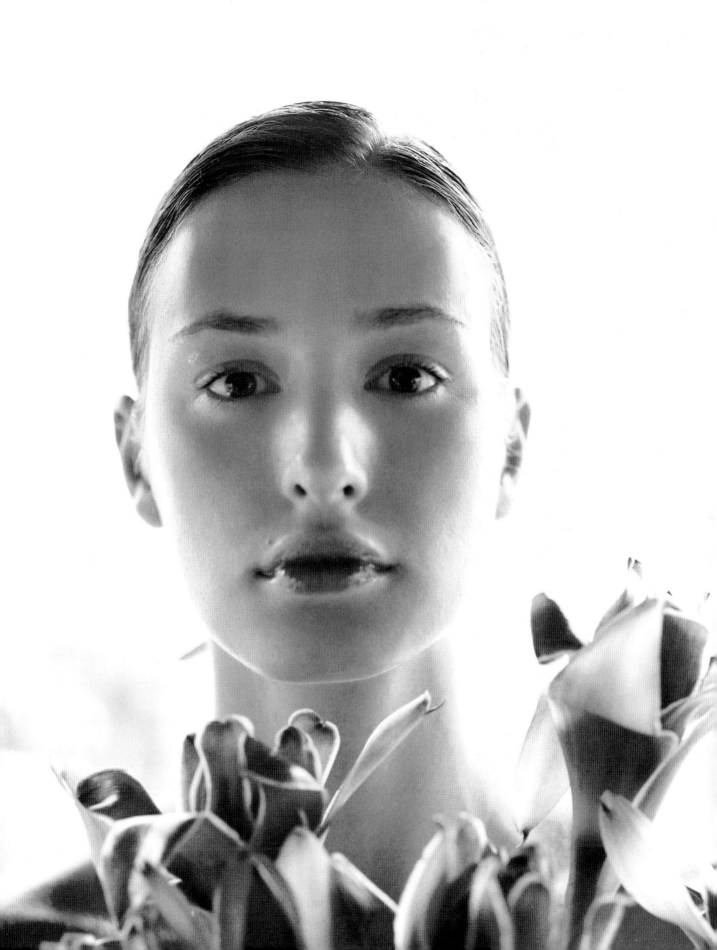

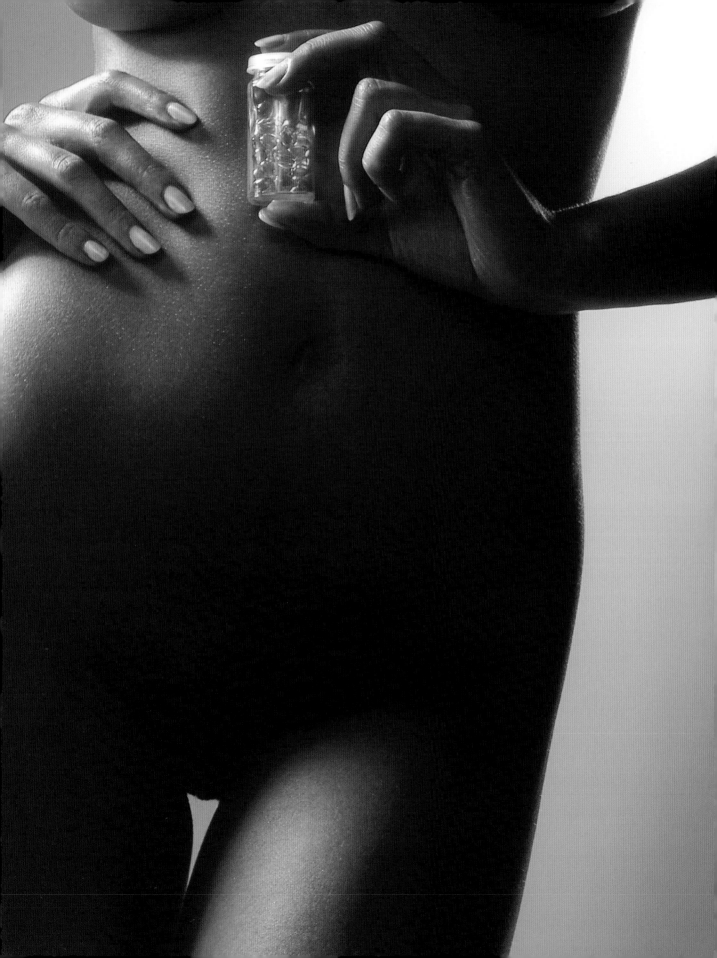

Complementary supplements

They're becoming more and more prominent as a way of recharging our batteries when dieting or to top up our intakes. Here are the stars in this field with, as a bonus, the foods they are found in without having to reach for the pills!

An antioxidant medication now being studied as a substitute for dietary supplements is already proving effective on animals. Meanwhile, these are the frontrunners for us.

C AND E, THE 'LIFE AMINES'

Vitamin C We are unable to make it ourselves and yet it is essential for fighting infections and degenerative diseases (found in blueberry, blackcurrant, parsley, citrus fruits, kiwi fruit, capsicum, cauliflower and red cabbage).

Vitamin E It slows down the skin-ageing process (found in wheatgerm oil, soy oil, walnut or olive oil, grains and cereals, oily fish, almonds and hazelnuts). One vitamin E molecule is said to inhibit the peroxidation of a thousand polyunsaturated fatty acid molecules.

POWER COUPLE AGAINST WEAR-AND-TEAR: SELENIUM AND ZINC

Selenium The enzyme that contributes to the stabilisation of keratin molecules within the skin and protects against the toxicity of UVA rays (found in oysters, eggs, mushrooms, chicken, carrots). Its effectiveness is enhanced when it is partnered with vitamin E.

Zinc participates in the synthesis of collagen (like manganese) and elastin (found in oysters, meats, wholegrains, lentils, oily fish, walnuts, hazelnuts). It stimulates immunity and improves certain skin problems, including psoriasis and acne.

• **Choose natural formulas** (read the label): synthetic formulas are not as well absorbed.

• **Warning: iron and copper**, notorious pro-oxidants, are strictly reserved for medically prescribed use.

THE WORD FROM PROFESSOR MARIE-THÉRÈSE LECCIA

Antioxidants can be of benefit, as long as they are not taken in a haphazard way: it's essential to be well informed and, above all, to take a complex of several antioxidants with complementary—rather than overlapping—benefits.

A short-term (three-week) course before a period of sun exposure is not, in principle, dangerous. But it is not recommended to take them for months at a time, especially if you have a balanced diet! Some women take them continuously—for fitness, a flat stomach or thin legs, and it's most often the same antioxidant molecules in all of the special supplements. However, if you have too many, they can become pro-oxidative and cause their own set of problems! This has been recently demonstrated by the results of a French study.

Anti-stress anti-fatigue

Managing your energy by rationing your emotional and physiological engines is also a matter of a tailor-made diet and carefully calculated nudges in the right direction.

Certain plants can help to regulate our appetite for ageing well.

Guarana, a physical and intellectual stimulant, slows down the emptying of the stomach and helps to 'burn' fats. **Caralluma** regulates the feeling of fullness, stimulates the basal metabolism and calms down behavioural food issues such as compulsive eating.

THE WORD FROM THE EXPERT Stimulants are false pick-me-ups! Coffee and tea, like alcoholic drinks, do nothing but enervate us and increase the excitability of our muscles.

MAGNESIUM: OPTIMUM

An element in the transformation of energy, involved in over 300 biochemical reactions, it is essential for our neurological and muscular balance. However, **stress drains our reserves** of magnesium ... Magnesium deficiencies are the first cause of feelings of fatigue. The foods highest in magnesium are fresh and especially dried fruits and vegetables, wholegrains and cocoa. A supplement taken at the changeover of the seasons is recommended by many nutritionists.

SUGAR ATTRACTS SUGAR

and it's not the real fuel for energy...

Insulin is secreted by the pancreas to allow blood sugar to enter the cells. Elevated insulin levels accelerate the ageing process. So we come to the conclusion that we need to avoid sugar so we don't stimulate the secretion of insulin! This is true, but it's not so simple: the glycaemic index (GI) of a food (its ability to raise blood sugar levels) depends a great deal on the other components of a meal. And highly refined foods—white bread, instant mashed potato—turn out to be hyperglycemic. Give priority, therefore, to low-GI foods: high-fibre dry legumes, wholegrains and brown rice, integrated of course into varied, balanced and colourful meals ... It's a matter of not nibbling away at your health and youth in the form of sugary snacks.

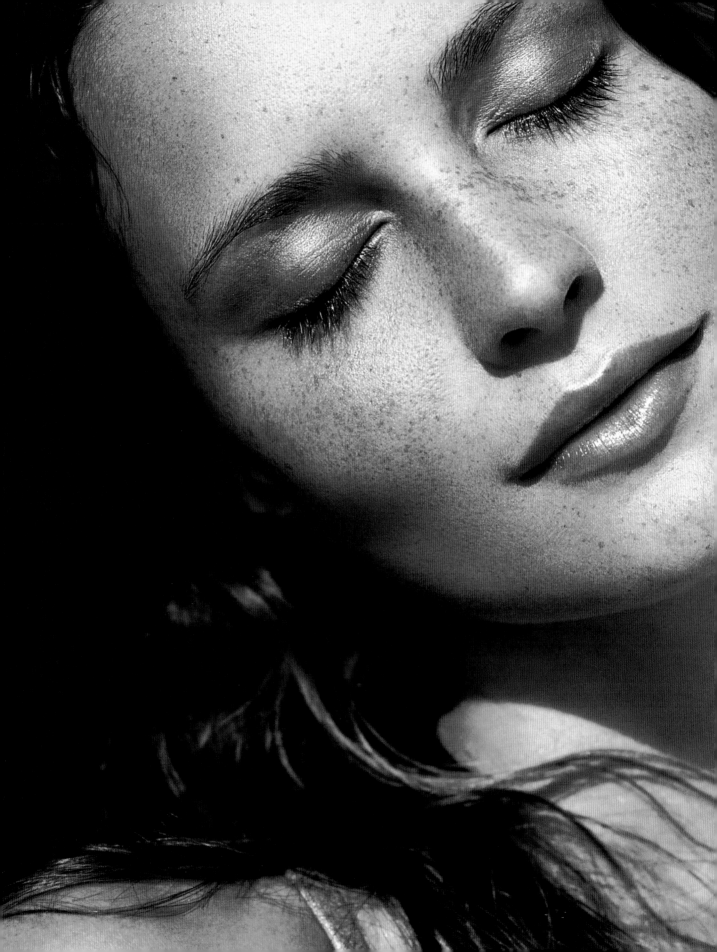

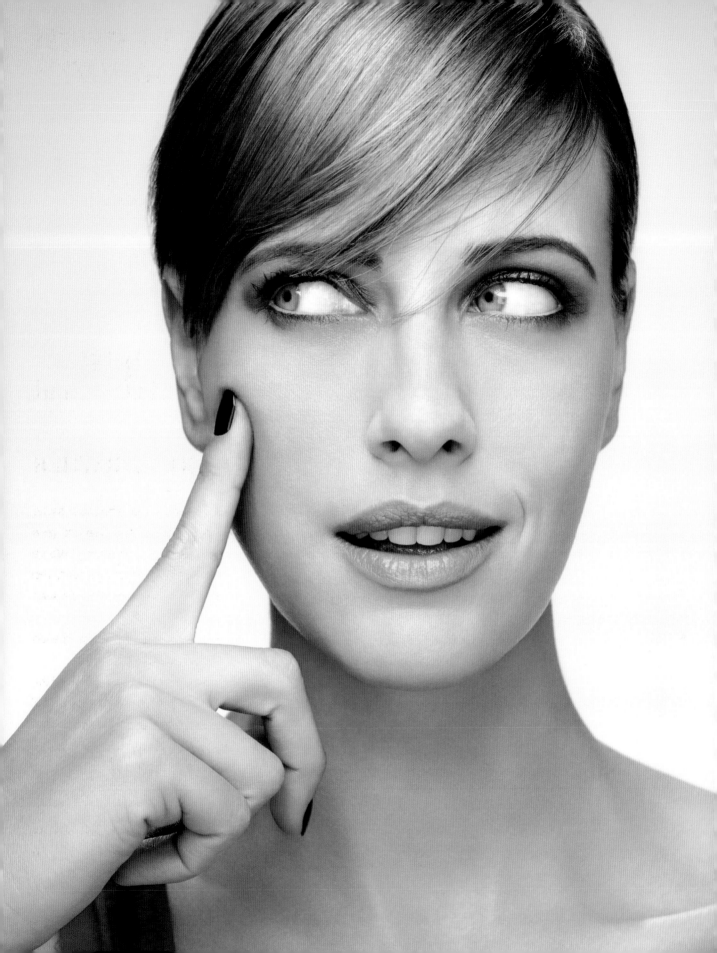

ADVICE FROM THE EXPERT: ANTI-AGEING TREATMENTS

Dr Marie-Thérèse Bousquet
Cosmetic Doctor

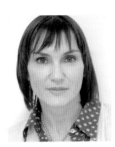

Marie-Thérèse Bousquet turned towards her area of specialisation very early on: cosmetic medicine. Based in Paris since 1993, she is passionate about the evolution of products and procedures offering ever more reassurance and wellbeing to her patients. Her expertise is the perfect accompaniment to Lierac's active phytocosmetic research program.

'It's **no longer** about fear of getting old but of saying **I am beautiful** ... and I **want** to stay beautiful!'

I PREFER TO TALK ABOUT A SOFTER LOOK ... RATHER THAN A YOUNGER ONE!

My philosophy is to have the individual woman understand, whatever her age, that she must make her peace with the passing years—and that cosmetic medicine is not a magic wand. We can give her real improvements, but we aren't going to give her the impossible ... an end to ageing! We've had our twenties, our thirties, our forties—I am coming up to fifty: it's possible to age *well*, the important thing is to accept it! I stress this point more and more in my initial consultations with patients. You mustn't delude the woman you have in front of you.

The practice of early intervention, even before the age of thirty in some cases, unquestionably makes it easier to accommodate the passing years, even if, of course, it can't suspend them.

I'm not going to indulge the patient who comes in with a magnifying mirror, saying: 'Look at this little wrinkle, it's terrible!' I want to guide them towards accepting things, which may seem paradoxical since my job is to fix whatever's troubling them. Without contradicting my profession, it is important to accept oneself. It's essential! I have a very wonderful job. It's very fulfilling to offer a new lease on life, happiness and reassurance to patients! The products and procedures available to us are constantly evolving, helping us to meet this challenge.

One can't, however, let oneself be influenced by the beauty standards of the day.

It's not desirable to produce clones. We need a few wrinkles for a natural, expressive face, be able to keep its mobility, its smile ...

▶

ANTI-AGEING TREATMENTS

▶We have to accept our little imperfections, reject the plastic surgery stereotype.

It's up to us, the cosmetic doctors, to approach each case, physiognomy by physiognomy, issue by issue—and refuse to support this disturbing increase that enters into a mad spiral. Otherwise it's a kind of hell, including psychologically.

ANTI-AGEING SOLUTIONS ... AGE BY AGE!
20–30 YEARS: HYDRATE AND GUARD ONE'S ASSETS

Skin texture, freshness, tone, it's all perfect. I just offer cosmetic advice, about health and lifestyle, by making women aware of the assets they have, which they should learn to preserve.

No cosmetic medical intervention is required, but on the other hand daily care is necessary.

The essential message is still protection (avoiding the sun, smoking). Current cosmetic treatments are nevertheless helping us to combat these harmful effects. It's obviously essential not to forget the daily routines like cleaning the skin, moisturising and having a healthy diet.

Simple and non-aggressive treatments, such as micro-dermabrasion or a glycolic peel, can be advantageous during this stage for refreshing the glow of a skin that has become dull.

Specific treatments Lierac's ultra-hydrating Hydra-Chrono line aims to remodel and boost the skin's irrigation system both on the surface and in depth using the Aqua Pump® complex, combining red microalgae and amino acids.

30–40 YEARS: HYDRATE AND STIMULATE

You start to glimpse little signs, the first indicators of slightly weakened skin, on a very superficial level, in particular the periorbital region (around the eye).

These tiny marks, which appear when you smile, signal the 'expression line' stage. Without resorting to injection treatments, cosmetic products designed to stimulate the skin are used.

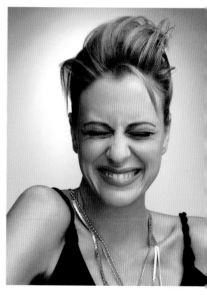

Specific treatments Lierac's Mésolift Concentrate boosts skin metabolism using an ultra-concentrated cocktail of vitamins, minerals and hyaluronic acid. There is also the Soins Peel (Peel Treatment), cosmetic peel treatments that stimulate cell renewal and hydrate the skin thanks to an innovative combination of alpha and beta hydroxy acids (salicylic and glycolic acid) and urea.

The famous botulinum toxin is being resorted to earlier and earlier to slow down the process ... We've discovered as a result that wrinkles are not only due to an alteration of the dermis, but also to repeated muscle contraction. Which explains the premature appearance of fine lines and wrinkles within the upper third of the face (forehead, crow's feet ...). This category of patient often associates cosmetic treatment with pleasure, the pleasure of

'Cosmetic treatments are more and more associated with pleasure, like using cosmetics'

enhancing the complexion, of having fuller, more defined lips … which can be compared to the practice of using cosmetics. It's not about fear of getting old, it's about the pleasure of affirming 'I am beautiful and I want to stay beautiful—and even to enhance my beauty!'

The physiological modifications of the skin make the appearance of these wrinkles natural. A gradual, quiet change: the thickening of the stratum corneum, loss of elasticity, diminishing of the dermis through atrophying of subcutaneous cell tissue (loss of fibroblasts and collagen fibres).

40–50 YEARS: ANTI-WRINKLE ACTION AND OPERATION FIRMNESS

The patients are getting younger! They are more and more assertive in their demands, especially 50-year-old women who don't want to look like their 70-year-old mothers …

The little smile lines are no longer as disturbing as they were at 20—on the contrary, they find them pretty, natural, a sign of expression. No, what they complain about is a tired look, contours that have

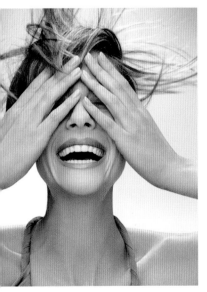

lost firmness, skin that has lost tone … just as for the rest of the body. The laws of gravity are unavoidable.

I am 48, and all of my childhood girlfriends, in the south of France, never thought about the question of their age until recently, and I'm not surprised to see them raising the question now. These women, who had never had concerns about skin ageing, are now knocking at the door …

Prevention is better than cure, but it's never too late to do some good. It's simply a matter of having appropriate expectations, and above all not promising to take off 20 years! Listening and offering wellbeing, a better life, is part of my role as a doctor. Those who began at 30, on the other hand, will, in a very gradual way, 'naturally' have this maintenance approach.

After undergoing a procedure, even a very small one, women regain their appetite for life, they feel rejuvenated. They are more cheerful and more attractive … This gets a certain energy going again—even if the effects of fatigue are there, the means are there for a return to form. Looking good channels positive messages—we must combat ageism but promote dynamism!

▶

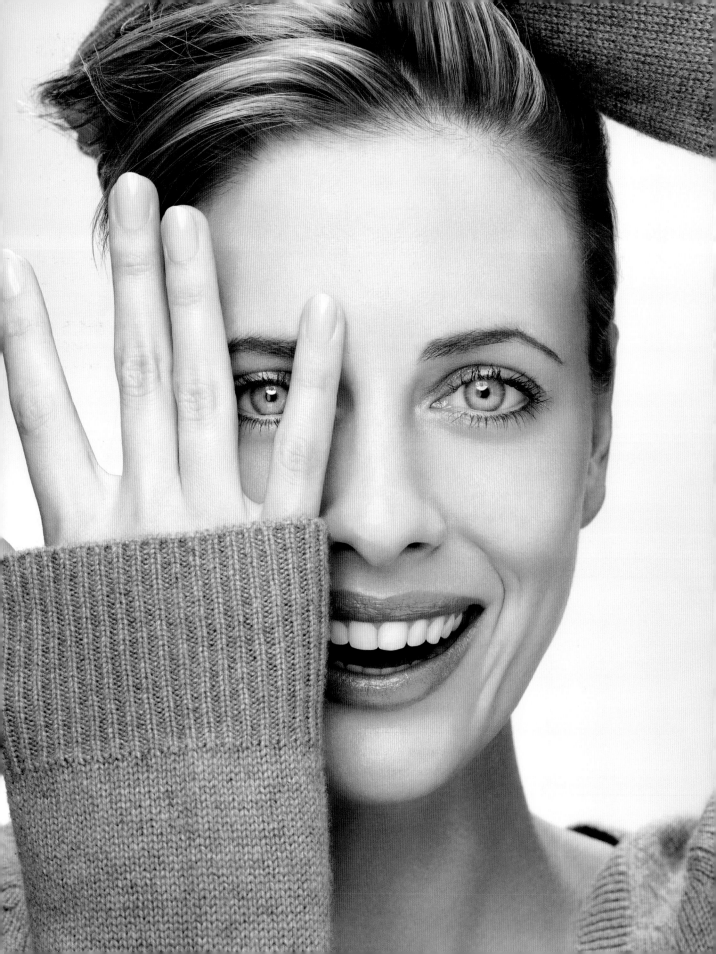

ANTI-AGEING TREATMENTS

'Even a tiny procedure can change behaviour, make us more cheerful and more attractive!'

Specialised treatments Lierac's Exclusive line containing the B-Relaxor Complex® has a filler-like action thanks to Génistéine®: a licorice leaf extract which stimulates the production of hyaluronic acid. It provides better hydration and prevents wrinkles, using a key skin-tensing effect, an immediate plumping effect, due to the supply of pure hyaluronic acid.

Cosmetics can prevent, stimulate, optimise and supply elements that nourish and preserve our assets—but they don't allow us to go back in time. When there is a loss of material, only supplying an actual electrical shock to the skin will restart the process. The cell will go on the defensive and start manufacturing elastin and collagen again—this is what happens when a burn heals.

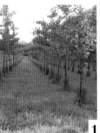 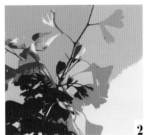 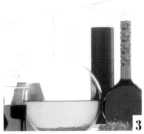 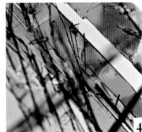 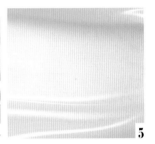

LIERAC'S PHYTO COSMÉTIQUE ACTIVE (ACTIVE PHYTOCOSMETICS) DEVELOPED BY THE ALÈS GROUP ... IN 5 STEPS. **1** A row of ginkgo bilobas in the arboretum. **2** Ginkgo leaves in close-up. **3** Extraction tests in the control laboratory. **4** An anti-free radical molecule. **5** A superlative texture, the crème de la crème!

THE WORD FROM THE LABORATORY
DOCTOR JEAN-CHRISTOPHE CHOULOT

Cosmetics are getting closer and closer to pharmaceuticals: an approach that comes from the source, since we find some very active substances in plants. At the same time that we establish the presence of active ingredients in optimal concentrations we also establish the absence of undesirable substances. Lierac has a **375-hectare arboretum**, and we are working on increasingly sophisticated extraction methods with the CNRS (National Scientific Research Centre). Controls allow us to check that there are no traces of pesticides. Modelling even allows us to restrict the harvesting period by concentrating on the 'good days': a plant will be at the maximum of its potential at a given moment, which it's a good idea to follow. When we process it, we only have a few days before us to extract the substance at the peak of its powers ... ▶

ANTI-AGEING TREATMENTS

'The most advanced research, including that on stem cells, can contribute a great deal to cosmetics!'

▶ADVICE FROM THE PHARMACIST: BRIGITTE LEROUX

The historical legitimacy of the Alès group in active phytocosmetics is illustrated by its **in-depth research on plant molecules, with patents taken out in conjunction with the CNRS, for example, based on rigorous studies**. The group is a pioneer in the use of plants in cosmetics, with a plant medicine laboratory and the first 'plant' patents going back to the 1970s. Procyanidols derived from grapeseed cuticles have been developed there since 1984, with an anti-free radical being perfected from 1987. It's the ultimate in phytotherapy, based on a demonstrated body of scientific evidence and a commitment expressed in a charter. Three hundred plants in the program (biodiversity at work!), ethics and cosmetic vigilance … with an ecological factory going back almost twenty years.

Under the guidance of toxicological experts, the raw materials are subjected to strict controls. A battery of clinical tests demonstrates the effectiveness of the products in totally independent laboratories or hospitals, sometimes using thousands of cases. In the same spirit, the Lierac Prize for Dermatological Research, awarded in partnership with the French Society of Dermatology, supports projects while at the same time allowing cosmetics to receive the benefits of the latest innovations in the medical world.

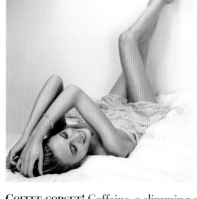

The active dermatological ingredients are perhaps the greatest step cosmetics has taken, with alpha and beta hydroxy acids (the new generations are even tolerated by sensitive skins.) Validated by the major medical organisations and the most advanced research: salicylic acid from the willow, glycolic acid from sugar cane, lactic acid found in tomato juice … Flavones and tannins, with major anti-ageing properties, stimulating the basic cells of the dermis, are widely used in our products.

COFFEE CORSET! Caffeine, a slimming champion, has always posed problems with its solubility: as a substance that's unpleasant to the touch, it wasn't possible to have concentration levels higher than 5%. Body Lift has succeeded in going up to 10% while keeping a perfect cosmetic finish, without alcohol or white marks … And Morphoslim acts directly on the fat cells, which it reprograms, via the stem cells, into cells able to generate firmness.

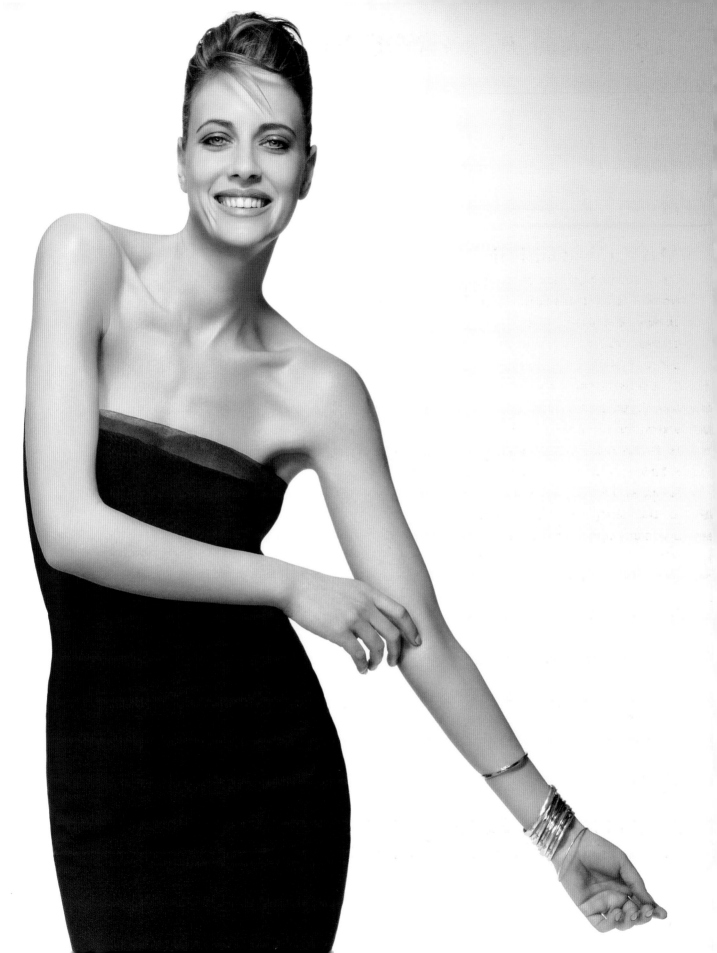

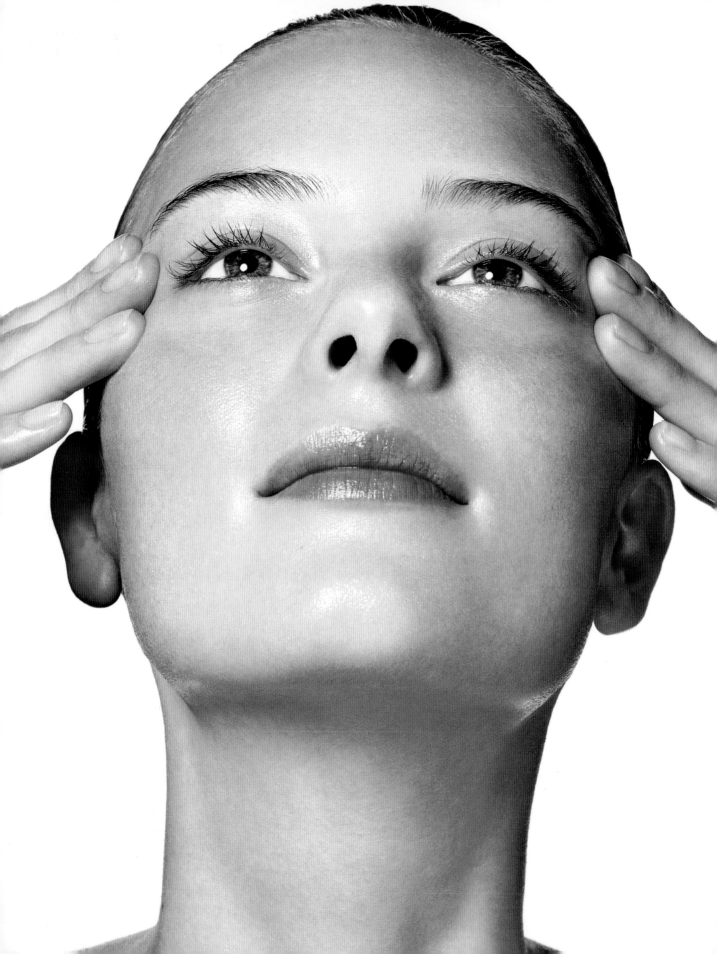

New-look technologies

The progress made in cosmetic medicine now lets us achieve natural results, a long way from the stereotypes of caricature and excess ...

FOR RADIANCE, action on the level of the complexion...

When the skin loses freshness, its overall quality is worked on by removing the dull, tired look—unlike filler treatments, it's the whole surface that's treated rather than a single zone.

These procedures stimulate the epidermis and the dermis: a more luminous, denser and firmer skin ... making a good look!

• **chemical peels** consist in removing layers of skin. The most superficial kind, based on fruit acids, stops at the stratum corneum. But the deeper kinds of peel, using trichloroacetic acid (TCA) and phenol, reach the dermal level. It's an exfoliation that burns the tissue: the chemical shock, felt even by the fibroblasts in the case of deep peels, boosts the synthesis of cells. Collagen and elastin fibres and hyaluronic acid hydrate and retighten the dermis. The microcirculation can be seen beneath taut, refined, clearer skin, resulting in a brighter complexion ... A really youthful boost, which in the phenol version can even smooth away lines.

• **intense pulsed light (IPL)** a procedure developed from the laser, with spectacular effects on age spots and skin ageing due to excess sun exposure, giving a more even tone and also boosting collagen production.

• **skin rejuvenation or mesolift**, a treatment using 'non-reticulated' hyaluronic acid or a mixture of hyaluronic acid, vitamins, amino acids and minerals which impregnates the surface level of the dermis and epidermis. The goal: to increase the skin's retention of water molecules (its hydrophilic properties), especially recommended for the cheeks, décolletage, hands ...

• **radio frequency stimulation**, which boosts collagen.

THE WORD FROM THE COSMETIC DOCTOR
Hormone therapy will maintain this elasticity—by supplementing internal stimulation with the anti-free radicals provided by the oestroprogestatives in gel or capsule form, ▶ obtained under medical prescription.

ANTI-AGEING TREATMENTS

▶ **FOR TONE, action on the structural level** to combat the sagging of tissue when faces become less youthful, with less defined contours and less prominent cheekbones.

• **injections** reposition the volumes of the face by filling.

• **thermage**: a new technology using unipolar radiofrequencies, which 'transforms' the tissue using temperature to create new collagen fibre stocks. A way of treating sagging without going down the surgical path—even if we can't see patients through to the end of their life without this being considered. The skin is firmer, with better tone.

• **thread-lifting**: used by certain practitioners to treat sagging.

SURGICAL OPTIONS (lipofilling): the face is remodelled using autografts of fat cells.

ANTI-WRINKLE OPTIONS, ful-filled!

Here again, it is a matter of injecting filler products, which are reabsorbable (for increased safety), more natural since they're more flexible, and are implanted smoothly (nasogenian crease, area around the mouth, between the eyebrows, crow's feet). A treatment that needs to be kept up over time, evolving over the course of the years.

• **hyaluronic acid** puts a positive balance in the skin's hydration account by retaining the water it contains, which diminishes over the years. Injecting it gives back volume and compensates for weakness in the skin. It gradually fades over time (9 to 12 months).

• it also compensates for the loss of natural collagen, whose consistency breaks down over time, allowing lines and wrinkles to appear.

• **calcium hydroxyapatite**, a new concept in filling procedures, restores the face by increasing the soft hypodermic tissue.

THE WORD FROM THE LAB
Collagen-based injections are now cultivated under controlled laboratory conditions (human or pig stem cells) and are 'bio' or 'dermo' compatible, without requiring a test beforehand. The effects last 6 to 12 months.

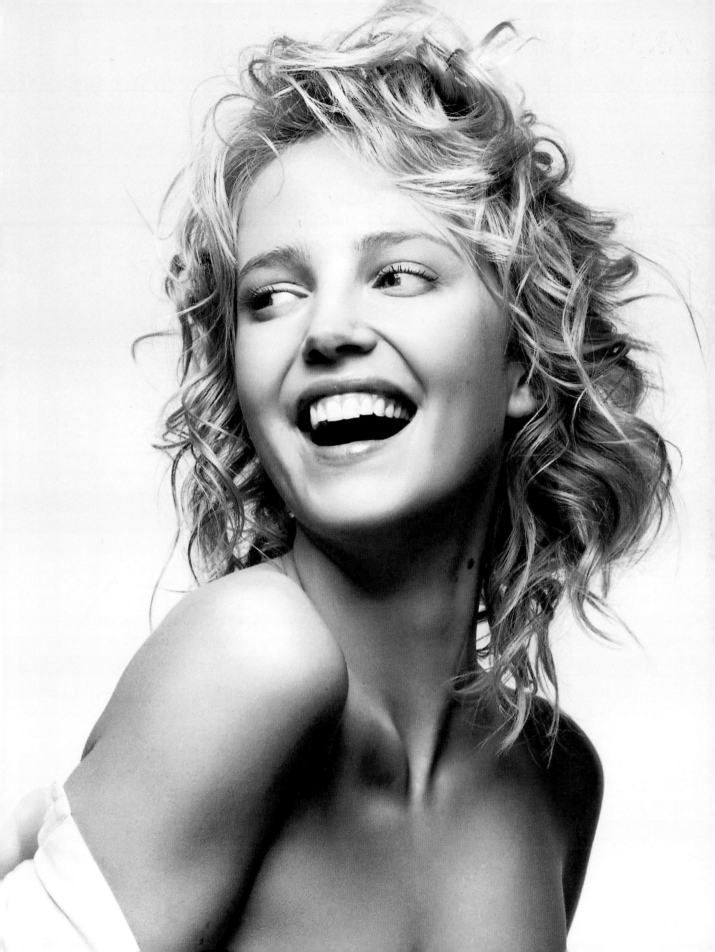

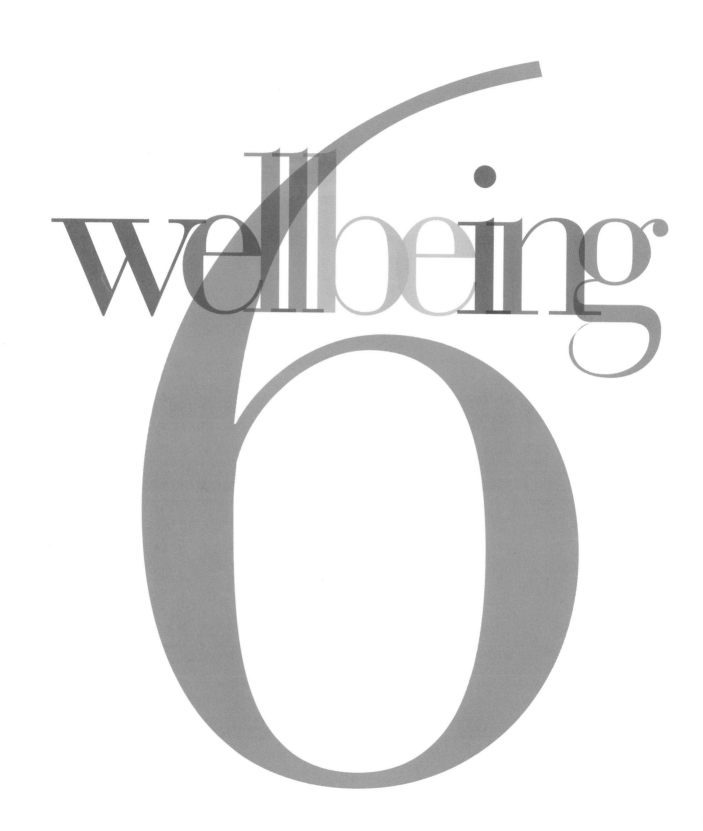

wellbeing

6

OASES IN THE EVERYDAY

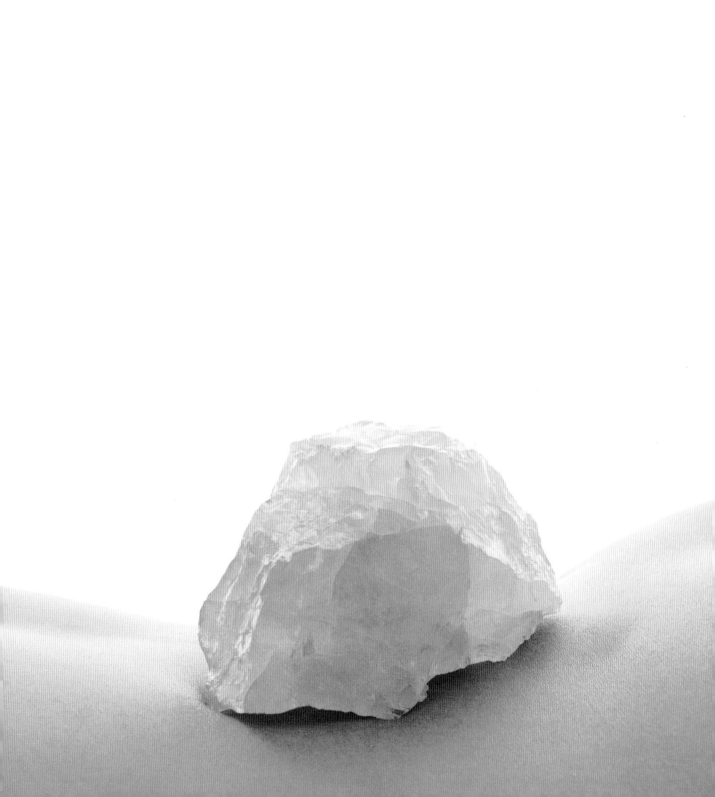

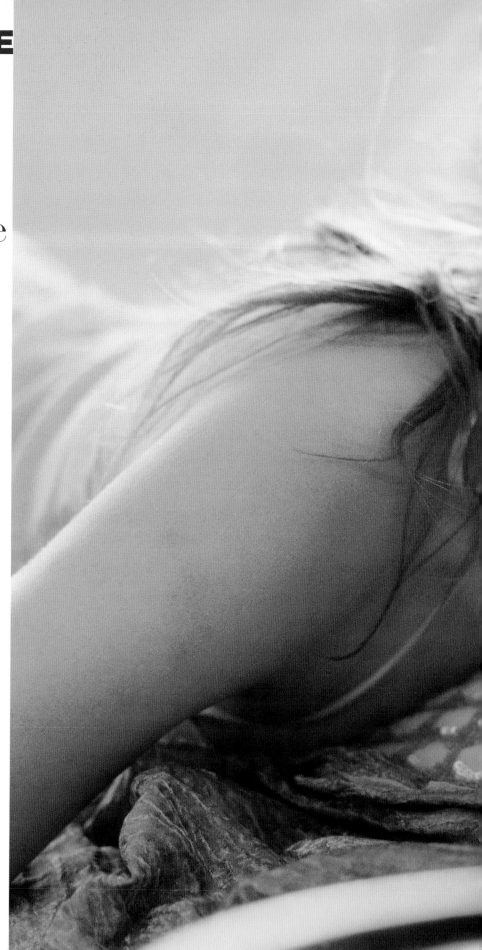

OASES IN THE EVERYDAY

Managing time now so you manage when it passes

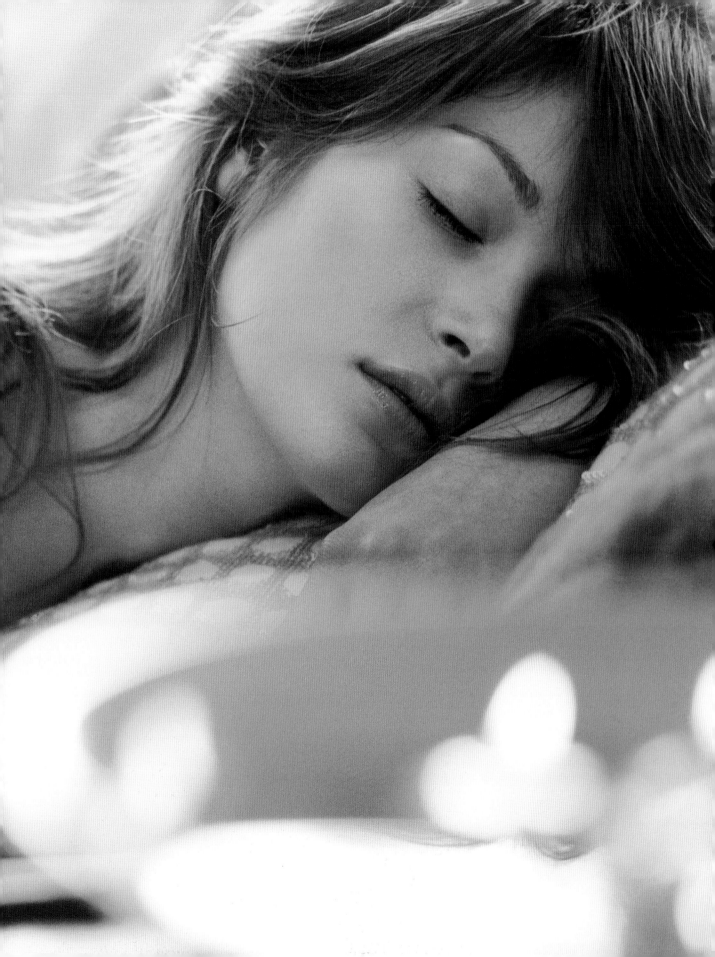

Chronobiology
about time!

Understanding your biological rhythms? It's ideal for getting the most out of your day, even if you're immersed in an intense work or family environment …

ON TOP … OF MY BODY CLOCK

Our whole metabolism is governed by chronobiological rhythms, which the body obeys to the letter. The 'remote control' that coordinates all of our movements is in fact located close to the optical nerve, in the **hypothalamus**, which wakes up the organism at the first glimmers of daylight.

6 a.m. The production of **cortisol** gets under way, the fitness hormone that powers the brain.

7 a.m. Get into breakfast—there's no risk of overstocking on fuel, even complex carbohydrates will be used up easily!

10 a.m. The brain has digested breakfast, it's in command of all of its powers. You can remember everything.

11 a.m. Biological slump: the well-known feeling of emptiness is not just in your stomach.

12 noon Light lunch to avoid overloading on sugars and blocking the production of insulin.

2 p.m. The body enters 'siesta'—**cortisol** levels are at their lowest.

3 p.m. A privileged time for brain activity.

5 p.m. The cocktail hour favours all forms of physical (and sporting) activity; the highly 'emotive' **serotonin** is at its peak.

6 p.m. The temperature of the body drops half a degree, which leads to hunger … and tiredness.

10 p.m. Melatonin levels rise and lower levels of concentration, blood pressure and body temperature. How about taking advantage of this to end the day on a beautiful note?

THE WORD FROM THE EXPERT
Medications can be more effective depending on what time of the day they are taken.

Our days, like our nights, follow one-and-a-half hour cycles. There's no escaping the few minutes of vagueness between each phase.

Express pick-me-up: training yourself to take micro-naps allows you to keep up a hectic pace without flagging.

THE WORD FROM THE COACH
Putting on your gym, yoga or Qigong gear as soon as you wake up, before even taking a shower, is a good way of making yourself do a start-up exercise session (even if short).

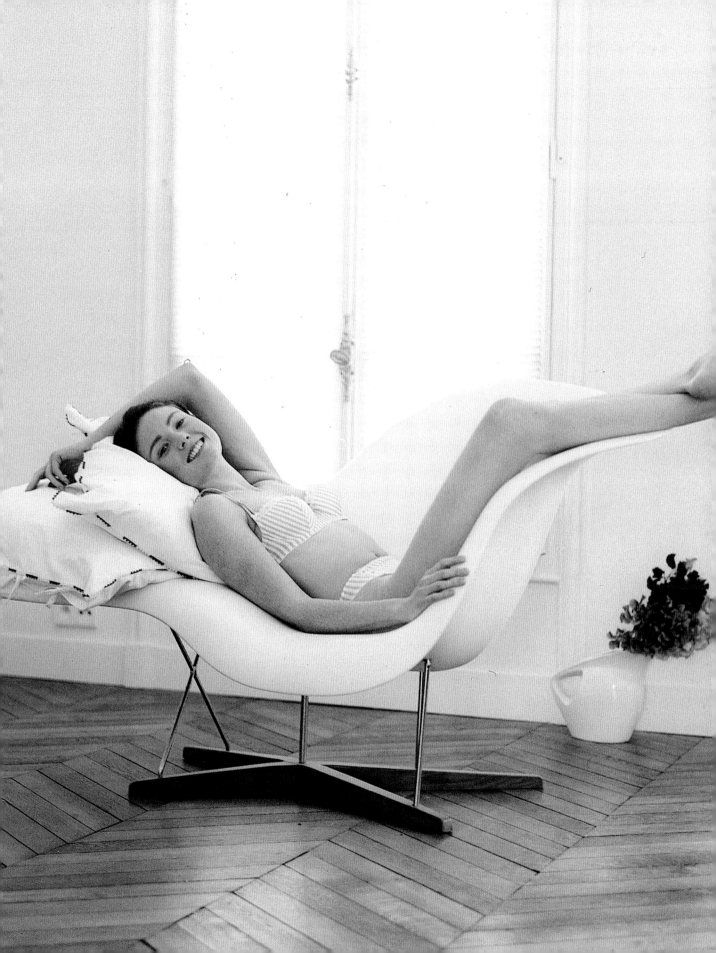

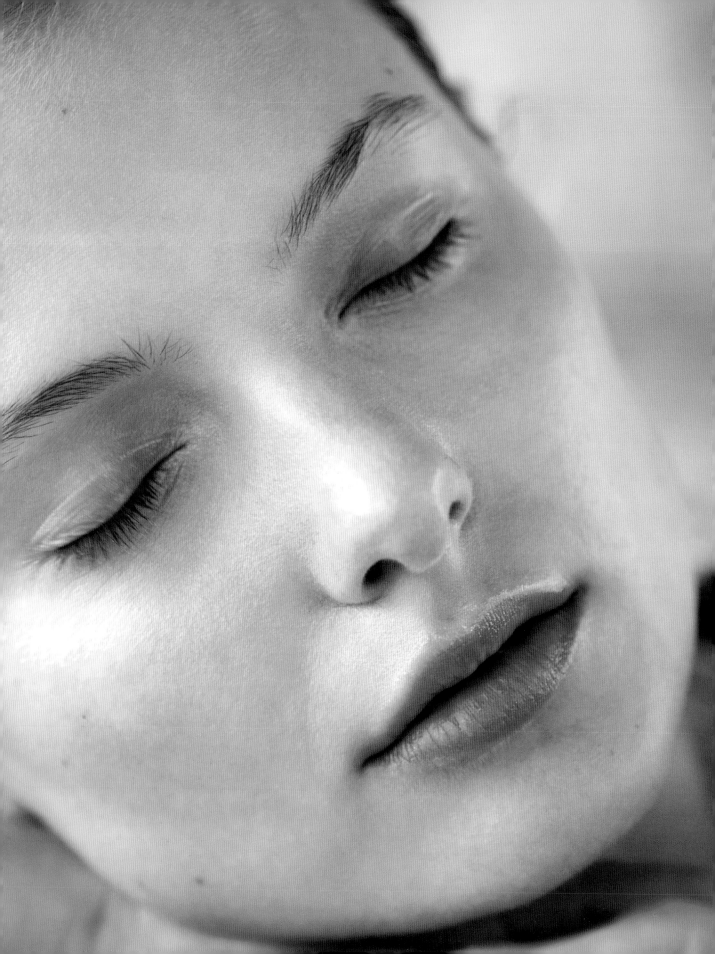

Deep sleep
good night

Work out your rhythms, manage them well to give your body a well-deserved rest. And give yourself the night of your dreams.

When we talk about getting our 'beauty sleep', it's not just an expression. The skin cells function according to a circadian (24-hour) rhythm, going from a defensive mode in the daytime to a **repair mode** at night, taking advantage of this time to regenerate themselves. Hence the problems connected to changing time zones!

LISTENING TO MY CYCLES

The physiological signs don't lie: heavy eyelids, excessive **yawning** are the warning signs that you're about to fall sleep. And going to bed too late can prevent you from sleeping!

Gentle strategies for gorgeous nights The later the hour, the more the body's temperature needs to drop: a **lukewarm bath** and a **herbal tea** (valerian, passionflower, linden) are the best form of preparation. Soften the lighting to allow **melatonin**, the bearer of sleep, to fully express itself.

The right amount of sleep From 5 to 9 hours for 'good' sleepers, divided into 90-minute cycles. The idea is to wake up spontaneously at the end of a cycle … It's better to get up and give yourself a nap later than to force yourself back to sleep.

NAPS: SMART OR SLACK?

A luxury for the body, which can recharge itself in just a handful of minutes if you've developed the art of the micro-nap, or in 20 to 30 minutes if you have a bit more time. It rids the body of tensions, assists digestion and ensures a good night. To be avoided: the overlong nap, which is difficult to wake up from and which takes you to the REM stage of sleep (dreaming sleep).

Overheated rooms are the worst enemy of a good night's sleep. Warm feet are fine, but keep a cool head: 18° maximum.
In one night:
• you lose 400 ml of sweat
• you change position 30 to 40 times.
Banish green plants, which steal our oxygen, and appliances that emit electromagnetic waves, such as televisions.
A good thing too—the bed should be reserved exclusively for sleep or love.
Anti-insomnia tip Putting on socks and gloves lowers the temperature of the rest of the body … and predisposes it to sleep.

De-stress
head first

Give your features a holiday in a few minutes:
four massages which eliminate the all-too visible tensions.

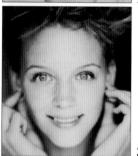

1

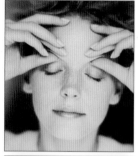

2

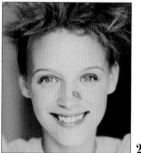

3

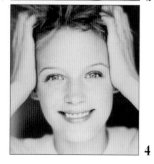

4

You can read stress on your face like an open book: if the nerve endings scattered throughout the epidermis send messages to the brain about external threats, the neurons, via the neurotransmitters, transmit temporary upsets to the skin.

1 **TIRED EYES** Pinch the eyebrows between the thumb and forefinger, applying a series of small pressures, from the inside out towards the temples.

2 **TIGHT SCALP** Massage gently by running the fingers through the hair, from the roots to the tips.

3 **SELF-ACUPUNCTURE** Pull on the ear lobe, pinching it between thumb and forefinger.

4 **THROBBING TEMPLES** With your hands on your temples and your fingers in your hair, make circles with your palms, clockwise, then anticlockwise.

THE WORD FROM THE PHYSIO
Eye yoga and posturology: find your balance (in the literal sense) after a consultation!

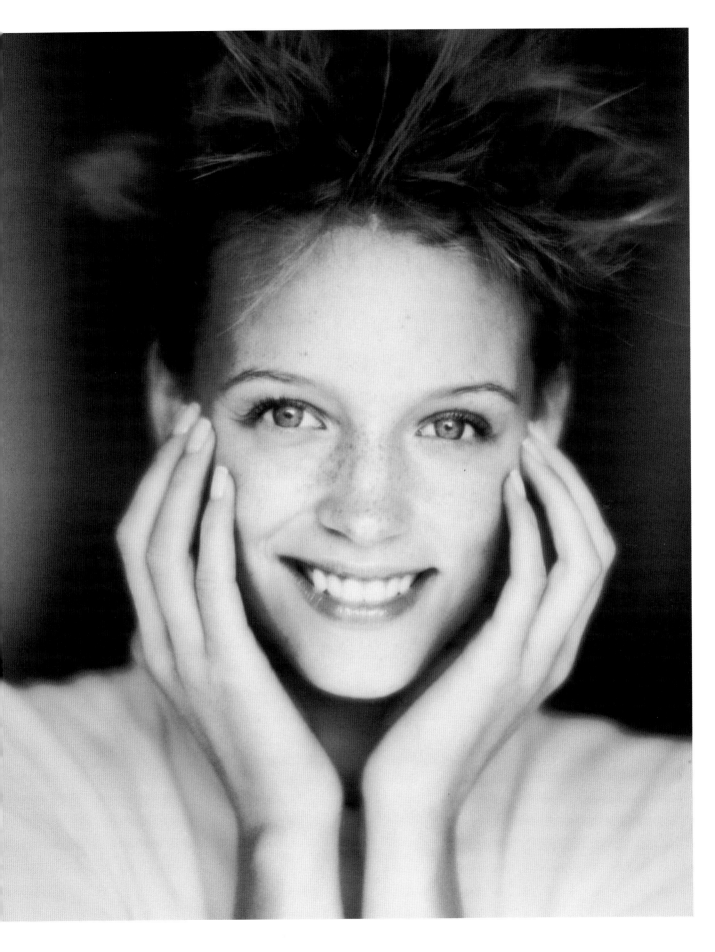

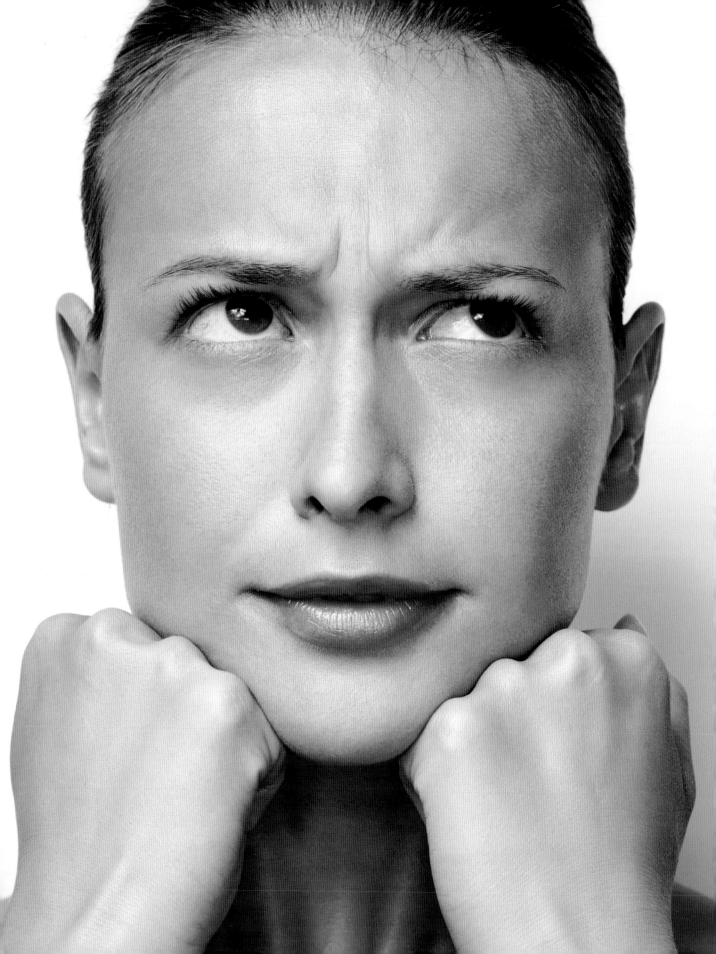

Face gym DIY facelift

Five clever exercises to perform daily:
a proven technique in the fight against gravity!

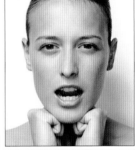

2

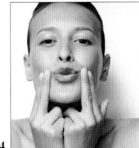

3

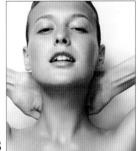

4

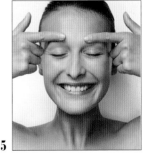

5

THE 5 MOVES THAT SAVE FACE!

The facial muscles are gently worked, without stretching the skin, by using the hands to offer resistance.

1 **OVAL OF THE FACE AND NECK** Mouth closed, elbows on the table, fists underneath the chin, try to open the mouth while working against this using your fists.

2 **NECK AND CHIN** Mouth open in the same position, the jaw has to prevent the fists from closing the mouth.

3 **NECK, CHEEKS AND INSIDE ARMS** Hands crossed behind the neck, push the head forward with the hands and try to resist by pushing in the opposite direction.

4 **LIPS AND AROUND THE MOUTH** Mouth closed, place the index and middle fingers at each end of the mouth, pucker the lips as if for a kiss while working against it with the strength of the fingers.

5 **FROWN LINES** The index fingers placed firmly at the inside edge of the eyebrows, which are prevented from drawing together.

ADVICE FROM BÉATRICE BRAUN
Repeat each of the set of five exercises three times in a row, ideally holding the pose for thirty seconds, every day and even, if you can, morning and night.

OASES IN THE EVERYDAY

Yoga inner calm

The wellness instruction manual: whether you have two hours or just a few minutes of downtime, yoga is a good way of getting in touch with your inner self, even without going outside!

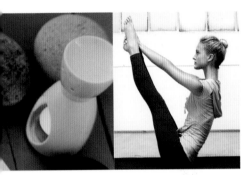

From the traditional **hatha yoga** to energetic versions customised for the West, all tastes are catered for. When Madonna, the most 'physical' of singers, strings *asanas* together in her dance choreography, it's proof that yoga offers benefits apart from inner peace. **A discipline practised for thousands of years**, yoga strengthens the mind while sculpting the figure at the same time; soothes tensions by restoring the harmony between body and mind; helps improve sleep; energises the muscles; makes the joints flexible, but also stimulates the internal organs. It has a preventative role for all of the vital functions. The **breath work** sends oxygen to the whole organism, speeding up its functions and boosting its energy while eliminating toxins at the same time ... including mental ones!

A power yoga posture balancing on the edge of the buttocks, back straight, toes pointed.

The lotus position
The meditation posture par excellence, it requires a very 'Indian'-style flexibility (and the help of your hands to place one foot on each thigh after another). Until you master this posture through practice, a cross-legged position, the tip of one foot inserted between thigh and calf on the opposite leg, back nice and straight, a flat cushion wedged under the buttocks, will do perfectly well.

A SALUTARY WAKE-UP: THE SALUTE TO THE SUN

1 Standing upright, hands together at chest level, raise the arms as high as possible, pulling towards the back and breathing deeply. **2** Bend the body forward, legs straight, hands to the ground on each side of the feet, head to the knees, breathing out completely. **3** Throw the left leg back, foot and knee on the ground, chin raised high and lungs empty. **4** Put back the right leg in turn, feet on the ground, make a 'plank', arms straight, breathing in deeply. **5** Bend the arms and place forehead, chest, knees and toes on the ground, breathing out. **6** Raise the head, pushing on the arms, breathing in deeply, pelvis and legs on the ground. **7** Without moving your hands or feet, pull yourself up into a triangle, buttocks in the air, lungs full, then bring the left leg forward. **8** Straighten the legs, hands on the ground, head to the knees. **9** Return to position 1 while breathing in.

▶

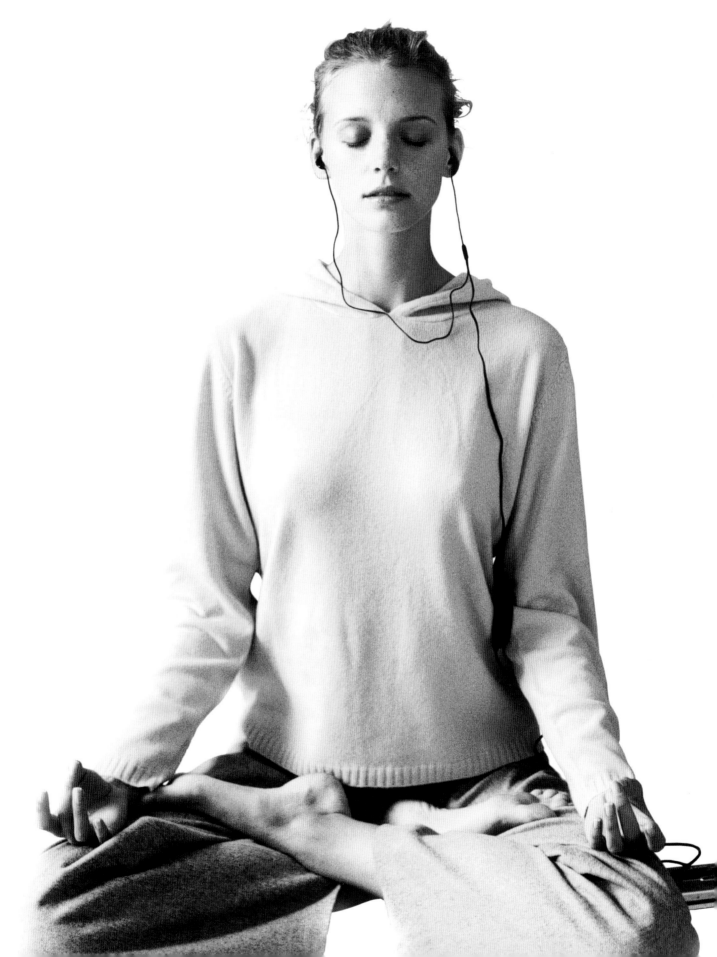

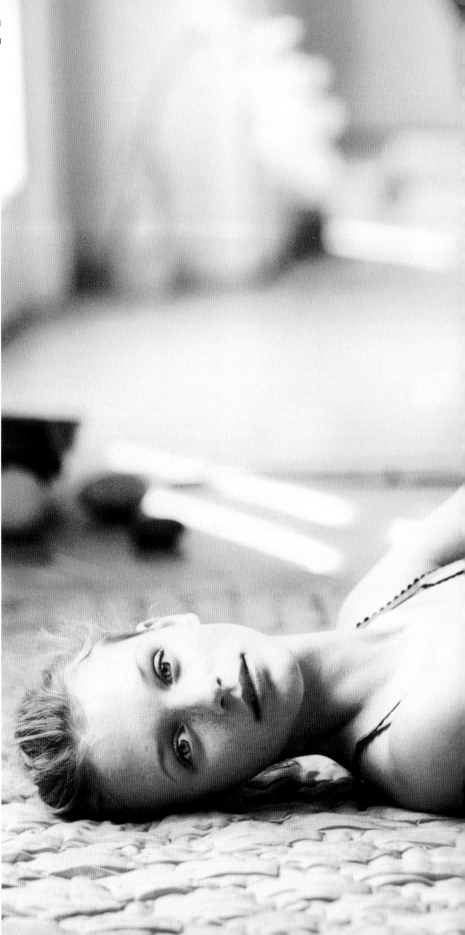

OASES IN THE EVERYDAY

YOGA LESSON
After the SALUTE TO THE SUN, stretch your back each morning with a series of simple movements: a very effective form of prevention against poor body postures.

THE BASIC POSTURE
Lie quite flat on a foam mat (or just a mat). Bend the knees up to the chest and hug them in your arms: for 5 to 15 minutes depending on the level of tension.

VARIATION 1 • Bring the bent legs right up to the forehead, exhaling fully. Lower back down slowly, uncurling the back and lifting the head off the ground.

VARIATION 2 • Bring the feet down to the ground, behind the head, legs straight.

VARIATION 3 • Bend the legs and place the knees on the ground, on each side beside the ears.

VARIATION 4 • Supporting the lower back with both hands, raise the straight legs to a vertical position, with the head aligned along the same axis, chin pulled in, and bend the legs when coming back down very slowly, always raising the head to soften the impact.

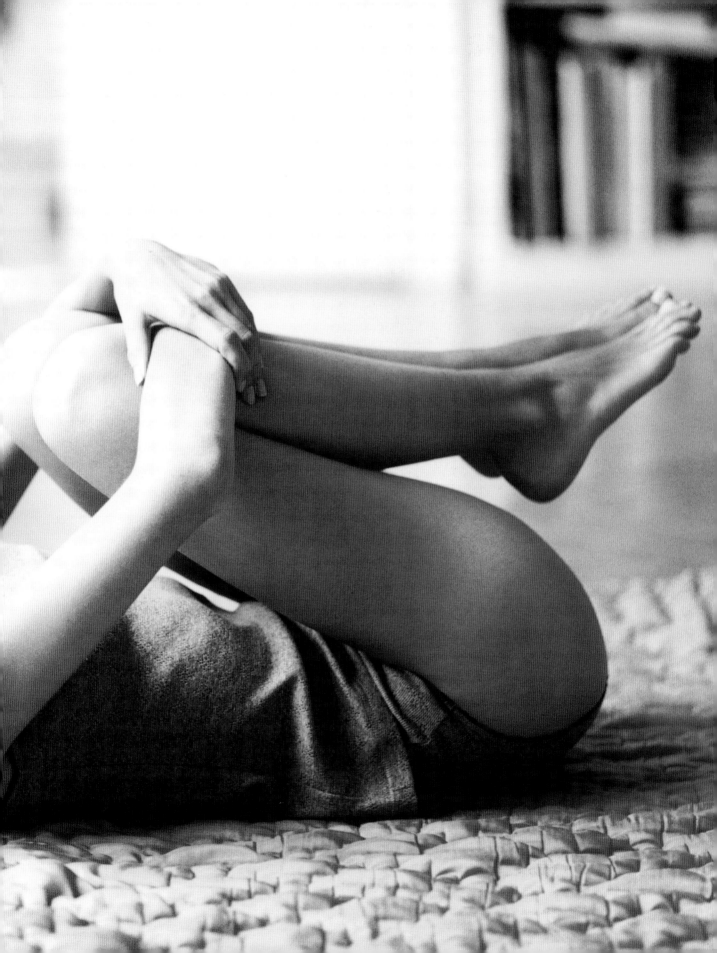

Qigong, Tai chi
concentrated benefits

Entirely oriental in background, these practices rebalance the energies with a very preventative approach, inspired by Chinese medicine and acupuncture. Have a teacher guide you, but there are no contra-indications here!

QIGONG: DETOX GYM

Slowness is raised to the level of a fine art in this 'energy work' inspired by Chinese medicine and Taoism, which works by restoring the flow of **life energy (qi)** throughout the whole body, through the use of meridians, as in acupuncture. A very gentle assortment of movements performed in a state of intense concentration, with breathing and massages that have a beneficial effect on the whole of the body, including the organs responsible for eliminating waste. And just the prospect of discovering **the 8 treasures** or of taking flight like a **purple swallow** is in itself a wonderful motivation …

TAI CHI CHUAN: RELAXED BOXING

Illuminating the shadowy areas of the ancient art of **shadow boxing**, Tai chi is an exciting reinvention of this martial art practised by Buddhist monks. Transformed into a slow exercise, an elegant rhythm of flowing movements, it gently tends to both mind and muscles. It leads to an increase in the powers of concentration, using extremely relaxing movements which stimulate the nervous system and blood circulation. With a current of warmth running through the body, you feel a real energy that helps you to overcome times of stress and overwork, with a feeling of wellness that gives you confidence in your own powers.

THE WORD FROM THE COACH
When you've just got out of bed, these are very harmonious ways to begin the day, based on the preventative quality provided by the control of energy flows.

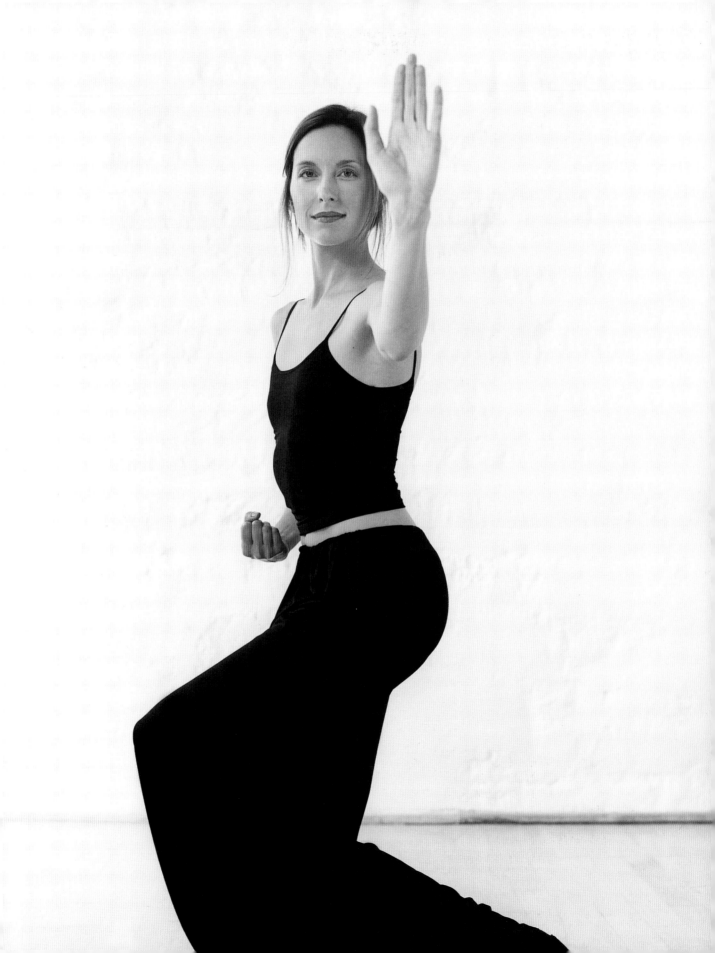

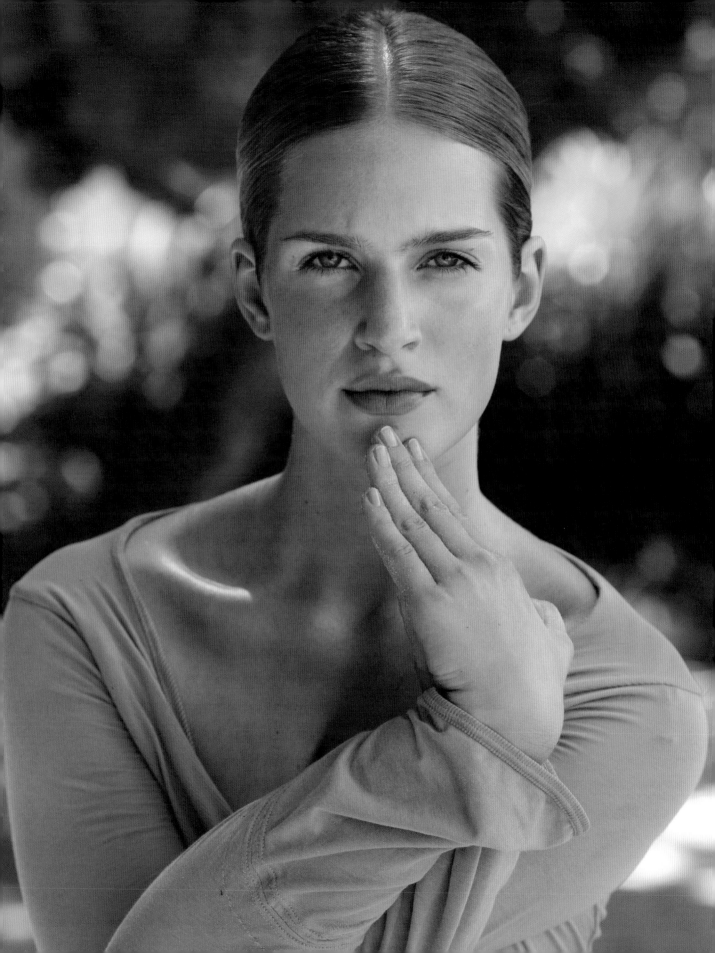

Gentle energy

Supple movements, filling up on oxygen without getting out of breath, a little lesson taking form ... without using force!

INSPIRED BY YOGA ... A short session of gentle stretching, to perform while breathing deeply

1 STRETCH The arms stretched on either side, the back nice and straight, lunge to the right side, bending the leg, then to the left.

2 UNWIND Back straight, pivot around: the left hand is placed on the left foot, then the right hand on the right foot. Then, the right hand is placed on the left foot and vice versa.

3 BEND Back straight, arms straight up and palms together by the sides of the head, bend to the right hand side, then to the left.

4 LOOSEN UP Seated, bend down towards the feet, which you grab hold of at toe level and straighten out the legs in front of you, leaning back on the buttocks.

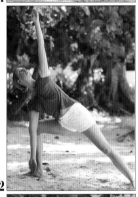

1

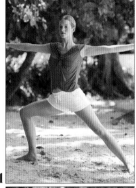

2

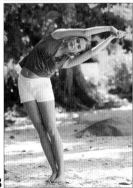

3

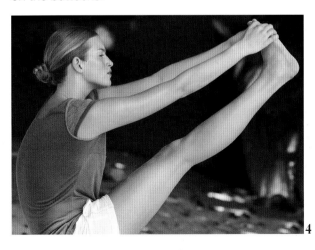

4

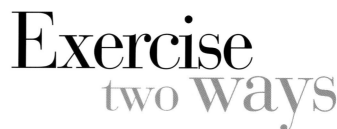

Exercise
two ways

No need for turquoise waters and endless beaches for daily practice of two dream sports: swimming and walking!

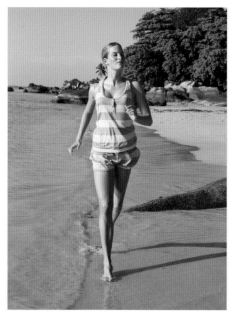

,LWAY COUNTY LIBRARIES

Wading at the top!
Ideally? In knee-deep water. Coolness plus massage, the effects of walking are combined with the benefits of seawater on the ankles and calves to achieve spectacular shapeliness.

ADVICE FROM THE ANGIOLOGIST
It's a public health issue! Moving is the best long-life insurance. Ten thousand steps per day is the ideal recommended dose for our body's faculties. Walking, swimming, cycling are perfect, but not all sports are good for the veins, such as jumping on the spot (step, aerobic) and static effort (overloaded body-building machines). Give priority to cardio training and exercises, go for doubles tennis and jogging on soft surfaces (5 km max).

SWIMMING IN BLISS

Swimming is the **royal road** to achieving the **body of a queen. Swimming burns four times more calories than running!** And as a bonus, there's no risk of hurting yourself: you're in a state of weightlessness, with no stress on the ligaments, you relieve the lower back, relearn good breathing, strengthen your cardiovascular fitness by boosting your circulation, as well as gaining the benefits of the whole body being massaged.

Each style of swimming has its specific qualities, to be chosen according to body type. Long muscles take centre stage. Toned arms (especially the triceps), developed torso, firmer chest, stronger back. **Freestyle** squares the shoulders, **breaststroke** develops the inner-thigh muscles, **sidestroke** slims the waist … and **backstroke** creates beautiful backs. Taking a few refresher classes is always worthwhile and will get you lengths ahead.

STEPPING OUT!

Seizing all opportunities to walk remains the best way to a healthy lifestyle (especially if you can't stand sport). Leaving the car behind or getting out one stop earlier is something everyone, including city dwellers, can do. Not only will it have a visible impact on your figure but, in addition, it improves the circulation, helps with digestion and elimination, feeds the body oxygen and slows down the threat of osteoporosis … As a bonus, a solitary stroll helps you focus the mind and make clear decisions. It's the simplest form of mental and psychological detox.

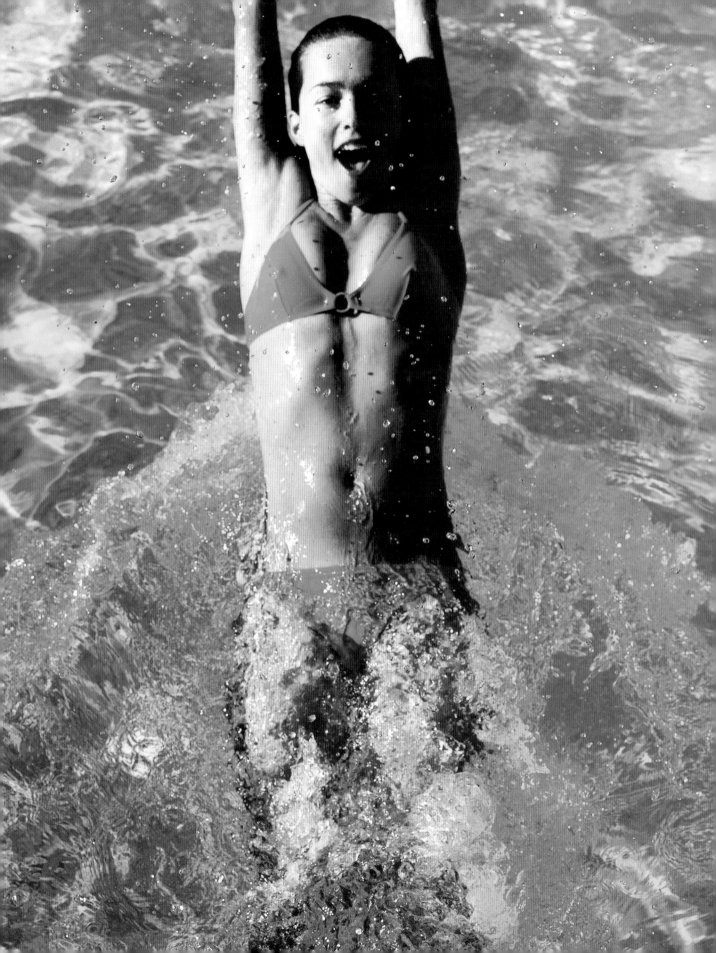

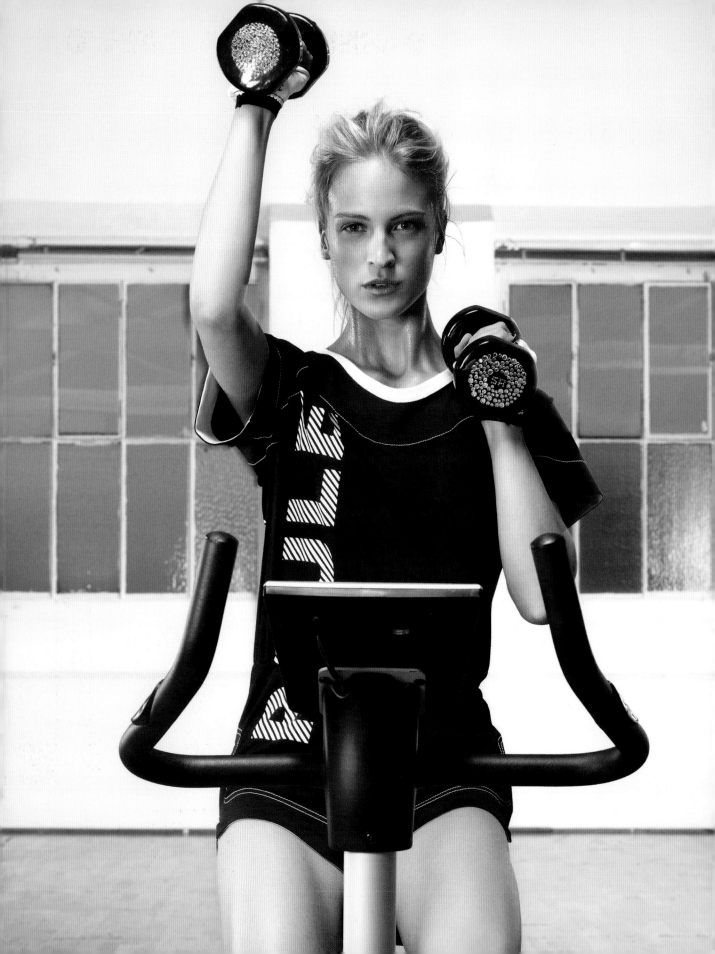

Body sculpture
gym sports

Invention is the order of the day! Machines are constantly offering innovative ways of carving out an athletic body for oneself and boosting morale for day-to-day demands.

1 CYCLING-CARDIO-WEIGHTS A very athletic combination: indoor cycling gives the cardiovascular side an intense workout, melting the thighs and buttocks. During a session which alternates top speeds with pauses to catch your breath, once the lower body is well warmed up, small weights complete the cardio effect by working out the arms without stopping pedalling, mobilising the dorsal, deltoid and tricep muscles.
Recommended if you don't mind getting your gym outfit wet …

2 SISMO: IT DOES (ALMOST) ALL THE WORK! A very appealing machine, since the oscillations it produces (virtually) replace muscular effort. A gyrating effect, from back to front and left to right (the motion is greater when the legs are further apart), mobilises the core muscles (which traditional body-building doesn't work out), stimulates blood and lymph circulation, and replaces, in 10 minutes, the equivalent of an hour of sporting activity. Four basic positions according to the targeted areas (in the photo, legs bent, for the thighs and calves).
Recommended if you're allergic to sport, or have problems with excess weight, back or joint problems.

▶

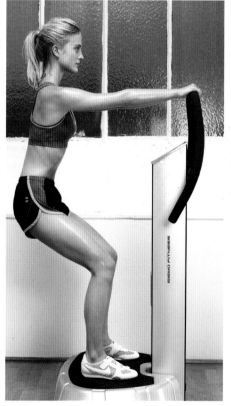

Toned, muscled, everything to give yourself a new lease of life and sculpt yourself teen-style abs.

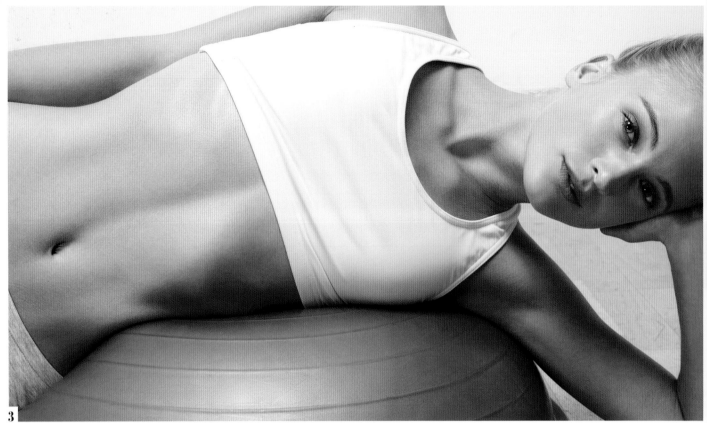

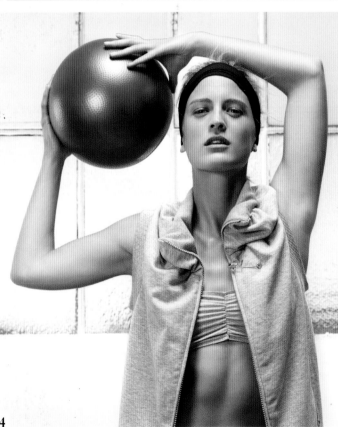

3 BOSU BALL: PLAYFUL Traditional floor exercises are transferred to this flexible hemisphere, which obliges you to compensate for the instability by mobilising the core muscles that support the abdomen and spinal column. Result: the waist is strengthened and slimmed. All good and lots of fun.

4 BODYVIVE: SOFT BALL Ideal for a gentle return to exercise, aimed at developing fitness, mobility, endurance and agility using accessorised sequences and choreographed moves. A customised program developed by the athlete Les Mills, the king of group exercise classes, with exercises varied using balls, elastic tubes and weights.

5 KRUMP: LET YOUR HAIR DOWN! The street dance revised and channelled indoors, for building concrete abs and buttocks while getting rid of your excess energy, or even aggression, to an ultra-fast hip-hop beat.

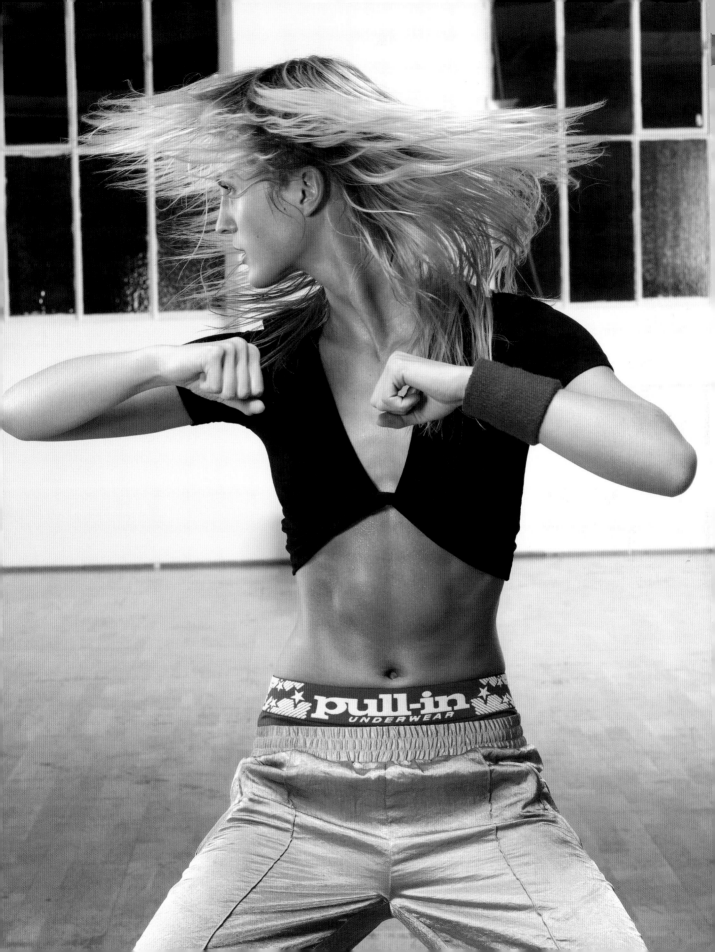

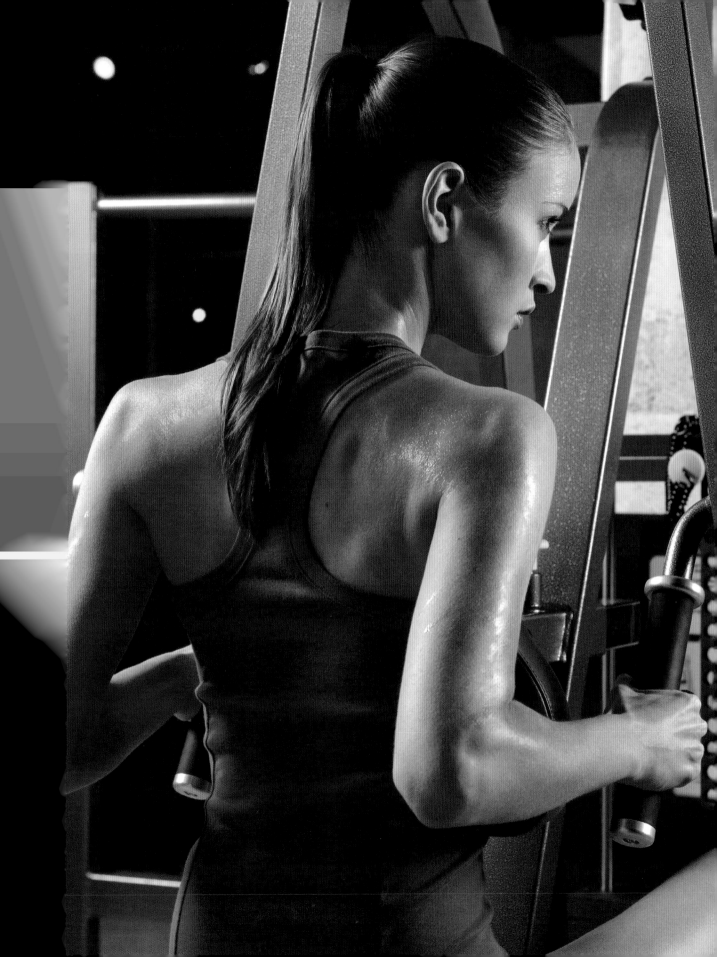

Body-building
taking on the machines

A feminine approach to body-building techniques
(but to be performed solely under professional supervision)
for ultra-targeted exercises. A guided tour.

1 MY BUTTOCKS LOVE IT They become incredibly firm in record time thanks to this machine, which works the large glutes without arching the back. Their curve is developed while slimming the top of the thighs at the same time. In a position on all fours, stomach supported and head in line with the back, the top of the leg is contracted by lifting it up towards the back to push back the bar. A technique reserved for true devotees of ab and buttock exercises, but which is in fact very effective.

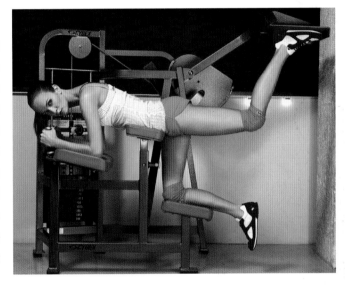

1

2 MY BACK ADORES IT Perfect for forgetting the hours spent in front of the computer, shoulders hunched and bad posture … The Row is a machine that works to open up the shoulders and develop the upper back muscles while at the same time improving posture. Seated back to front on a bench, push a bar out horizontally until your arms are straight. Well supported at chest level, you can feel the intense work of the muscles radiating out from the shoulder blades down the arms. To be used in moderation in case of problems with the neck bones, or shoulder pains.

THE WORD FROM THE COACH
Weight-room workouts have evolved a great deal and adapted to new expectations by becoming increasingly customisable: choosing an exercise ► should be made after thorough consultation with the pros who are there to point you in the right direction.

OASES IN THE EVERYDAY

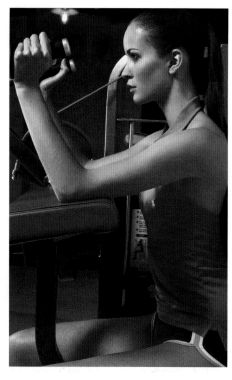

3

3 UP IN ARMS The abdominal belt locked, the back well supported, you lower the arm, breathing out, and raise it breathing in: a machine that allows you to sculpt the triceps (the back of the arms, which tends to betray us very early), as long as you perform long sets lifting a moderate amount of weight. A long-term project, and not one for 'cut' arms, using heavier loads and short sets …

4 FOR MELTING MY THIGHS The treadmill, star of cardio equipment (giving the lungs and heart a workout), redesigned in a inclined version to get the thighs and buttocks more involved (the steeper the slope, the more effective it is for developing muscle and losing fat), as long as you don't arch the back. The treadmill belt absorbs shock (the knees and ankles don't suffer), and the machine is adaptable to any age and physical condition.

5 THE BUTTERFLY EFFECT: IMPECCABLE PECS Pecs of steel are the greatest gift you can give to your décolletage. The Butterfly helps out by multiplying the effort you put in, arms apart, to bring the elbows together, moving like butterfly wings. The abs are blocked so that the arms work solo, not a straight-forward matter when you increase the weight: you feel it afterwards, but the results are worth it if you keep it up.

6 ROCK ABS For rediscovering your rectus abdominis (which singers know by heart) or your obliques, if you want to slim your waist. The chest leaning on the lever, abs clenched, you lean over until you're horizontal, by lowering a (moderate) load, and then raise yourself, breathing in, without jerking, maintaining constant control.

7 ANTI-SADDLEBAGS Burn fat and wake up muscles little used when you're a woman, the **abductors**, which extend the buttock muscles on the outside of the thighs, while gradually getting stronger. Seated, back and feet supported, the legs are pushed apart using the force of the thighs, without involving the torso.

THE WORD FROM
THE COACH
EXCESS KILOS,
NOT ENOUGH
EXERCISE
• cardio machines,
combined with a diet
program.
NO EXCESS KILOS,
BUT NO TONE
• weights machines
using moderate loads
and 15 minutes of
cardio to warm up.
THIN, BUT NOT
ENOUGH MUSCLE
• a warm-up, then
weights, with
gradually increasing
loads in short sets.
AND STRETCHING
FOR EVERYONE
at the end of the
workout!

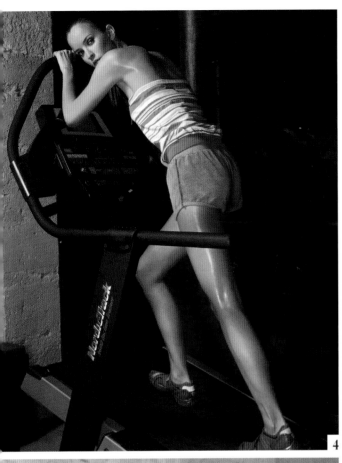

4

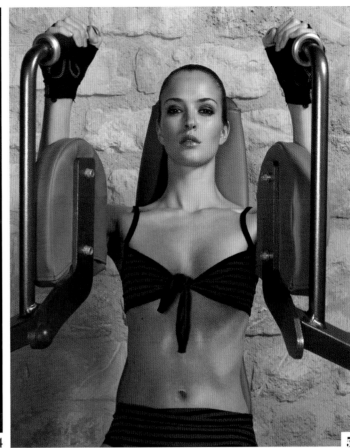

5

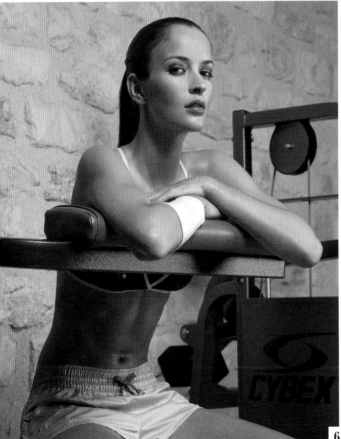

6

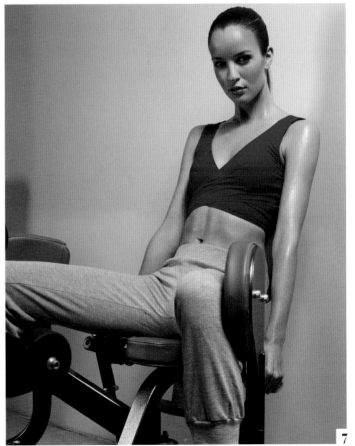

7

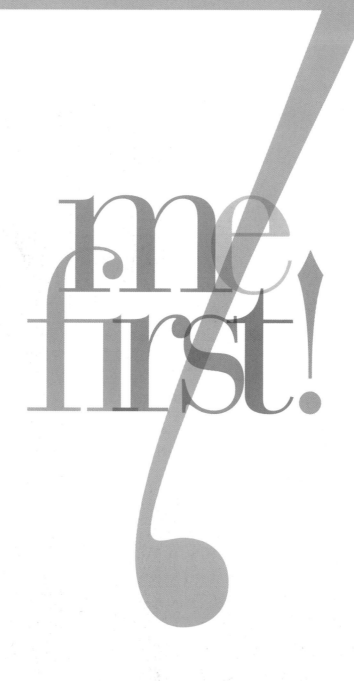

THE BEST OF THE WORLD

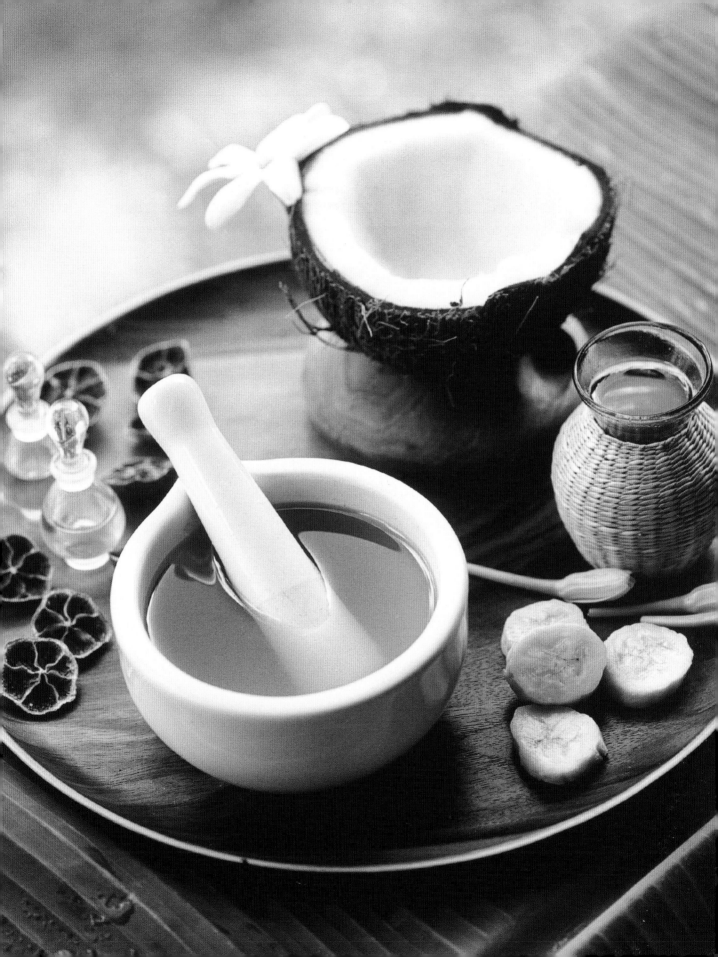

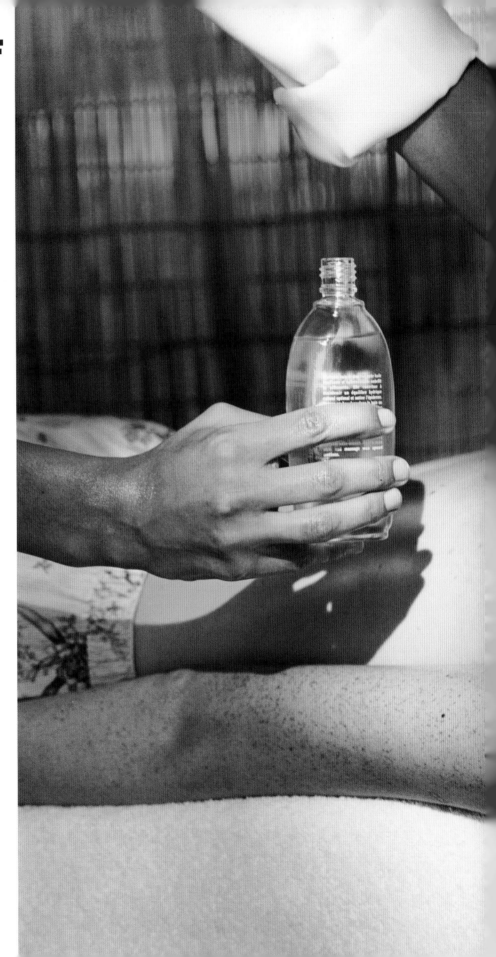

Rely on
relaxation
let go

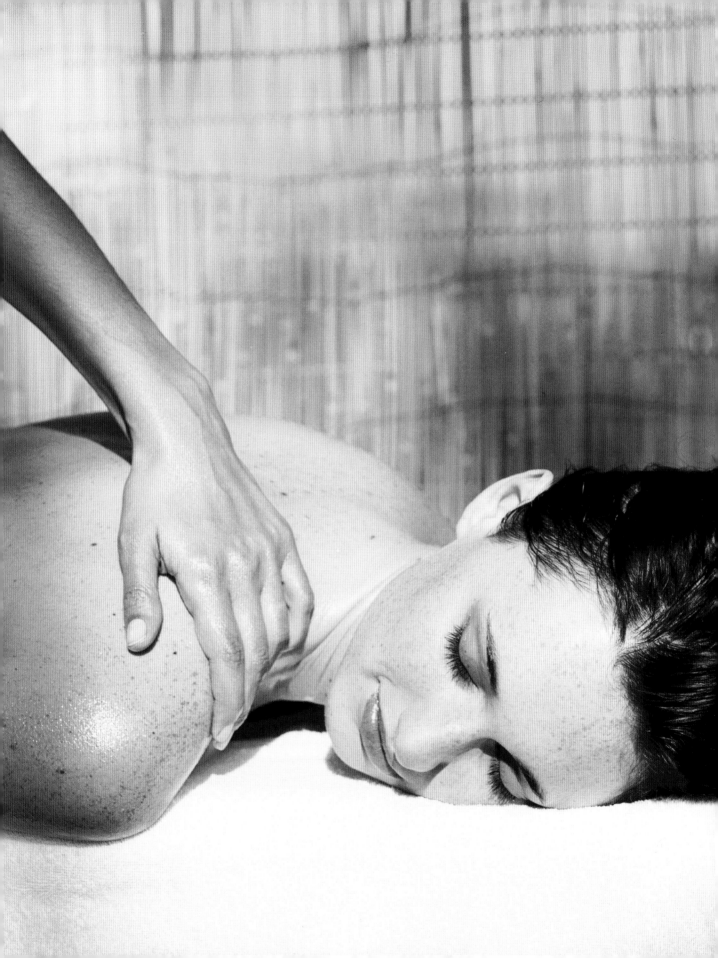

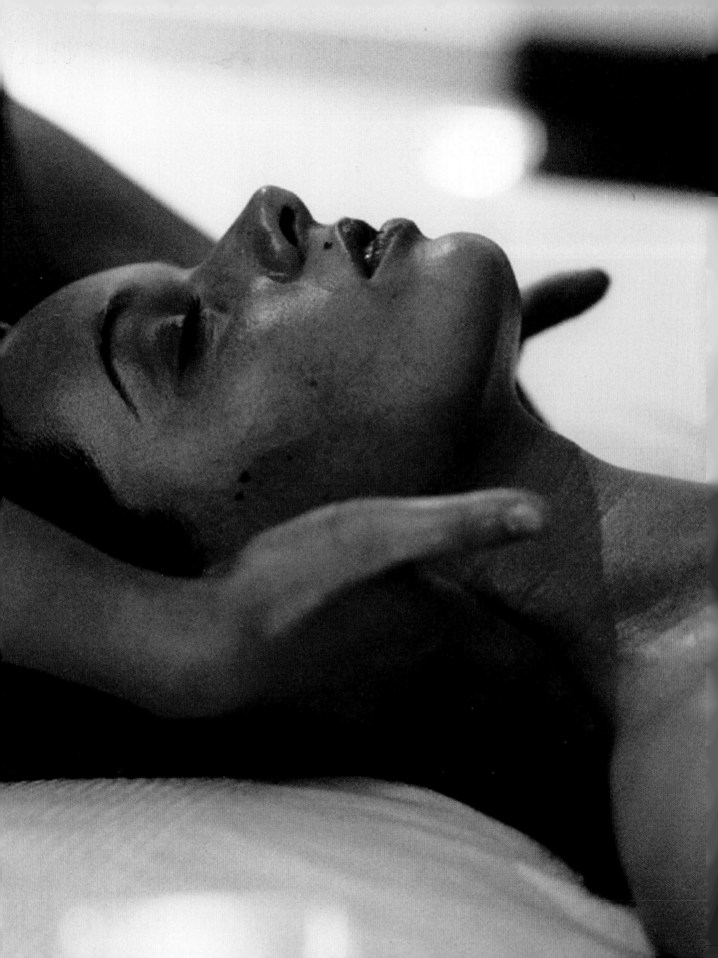

Massages:
in good hands

Kneading, stroking, palpating ... the culture of touch rehabilitated at last! Increasingly popular, manual therapies offer immediate comfort and lasting benefits. Making yourself feel good is increasingly recommended.

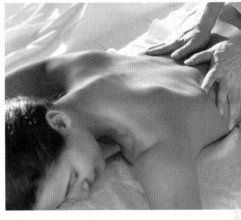

The decompression chamber par excellence, massage eliminates muscular and mental tensions, improves blood and lymphatic circulation (crucial for the immune system's defences), stimulates the nerve impulses, improves exchanges within the body, revives dysfunctional organs and soothes aches. Coming from civilisations where **tactility meets utility**, it immediately finds a means of communication: the language of the body is universal. By touching the skin, an incalculable number of **nerve endings** are woken up, directly in communication with the brain via neurotransmitters. A release of **adrenaline** (a stimulant) sends a concentrated dose of targeted pleasure to the brain, via **acetylcholine** (soothing) and **dopamine** (uplifting).

THE UNIVERSE OF MASSAGE

Ayurvedic massage forms part of the daily life of Indians from the cradle onwards: the harmony between the three elements (air, earth, fire) is restored using warm oils and sweeping movements. Japanese **Shiatsu** massage, acupressure, relaxing pressure applied to the meridians to rebalance the energies ... Native American-style **hot stone massage**, alternating hot (volcanic basalt) and cold (marble) on the meridian pathways. The languorous **Thai** massage ...

And Europe? The Greeks and Romans were acquainted with massage (thanks to the Chinese), Hippocrates recommended it ... and centuries of hypocrisy condemned it until a **Swedish** doctor, Pehr Henrik Ling, reinvented physical therapy in the nineteenth century. The re-conquest is under way.

FEELING THEIR WAY
The first European masseurs were blind, as modesty demanded!

BACK OFF, BACK PAIN!
Poor standing or sitting positions, pulling a muscle, chills, injuries or simple stress ... there are no lack of reasons for making an appointment.
A doctor can provide a prescription for a physio-massage therapist.
Or you might prefer the chiropractor or osteopath—each school has its adherents: the choice of the right manual therapy comes down to personal experience!

Happiness from the feet up

Following in the footsteps of reflexology, coming out of Chinese medicine, sophisticated massage or just comforting strokes, a supreme source of comfort … jump in feet first.

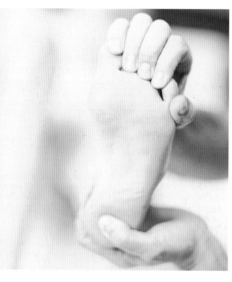

REFLEXOLOGY Good for the sole

In Chinese medicine, the arch of the foot sums up the whole body in **60 reflex points** (and **7200 nerve endings**), which the reflexologist will act on by applying pressure, in order to release the toxins that impede nerve impulses and vital energy. An alternative medicine that is both preventative and curative, though the Westernised approach gives more emphasis to the relaxation aspect: the proof being that you're supposed to come out of it … walking on air.

PASS ON THE MASSAGE

Enclosed in a hot prison, when the foot is released from its shoe and its every joint and toe gently manipulated, it will show you boundless gratitude!

Evening repair Massage from the outside towards the inside to relieve the arch of the feet and pamper weary heels, with the active support of a moisturising cream to ease stiffness and soften hard skin while preserving the hydrolipidic film.

SELF-MASSAGE IS GOOD … massaging with someone else

is better! Wellbeing, total relaxation, but also **sensuality** all come together. With a massage oil, for the pleasure of it.

GOOD REFLEXES

Keep a wooden foot massage roller with little spikes under the desk to roll your feet over, for relaxation in any situation.

THE WORD FROM THE REFLEXOLOGIST
Begin with the left foot, the 'Emperor's side', where toxins build up. The right foot, the 'Queen's side', is the seat of the emotions and deep energies. Stretching the toes lets you work on the brain, ears and eyes.

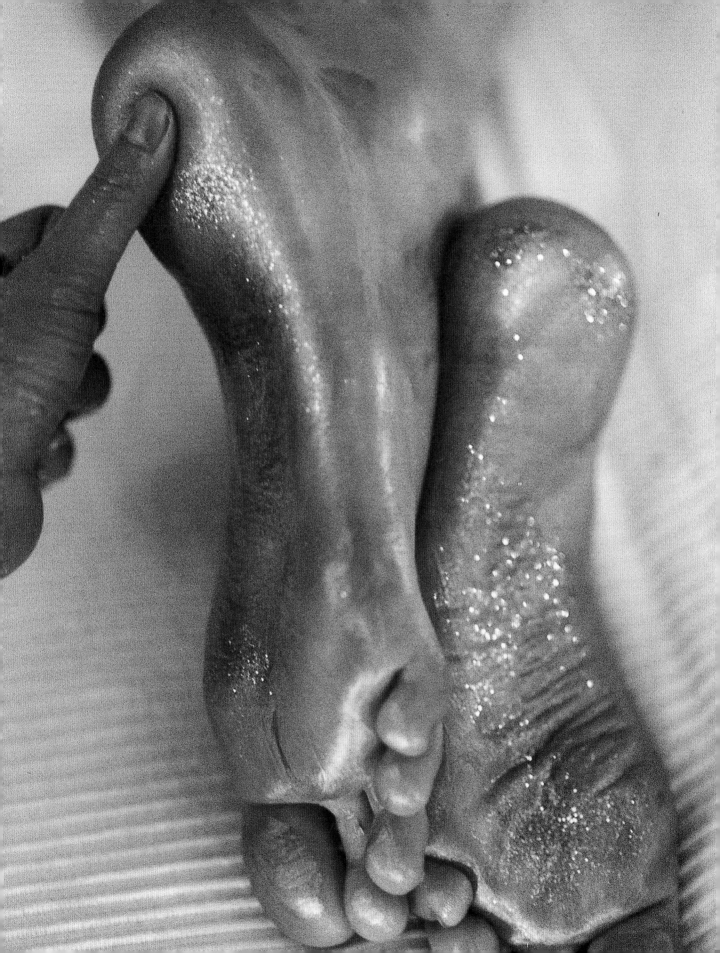

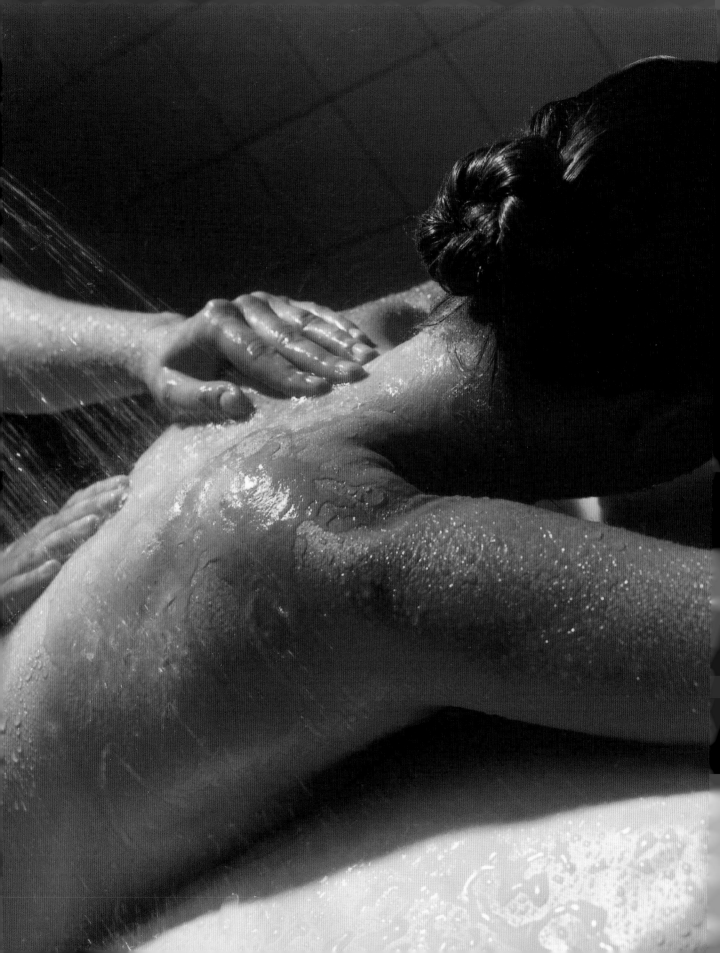

Thermal
dynamics

*It's possible to prescribe yourself happiness therapy.
The proof is in the countless thermal spring towns
whose health treatments are bundled up in pleasure packages.*

DIRECT FROM THE SOURCE

Take advantage of the fascinating resources of miraculous spring waters, energising muds and naturally therapeutic gases, which draw their incredible properties from the earth's core. A strict set of legislation protects their integrity and permanently scrutinises the consistency of their composition, up to about forty minerals and trace elements. Magnesium, typical of waters high in sodium chloride (Dax), sodium bicarbonate (Vichy), and calcium sulfate (Vittel) …

VITALITY MEDICINE

Beyond the idea of curing, the concept of wellbeing, which consists of optimising one's vital potential, fits thermal therapy like a glove. Prevention is the buzz word!

Wellbeing is enhanced when the benefits of the treatments are combined with a better dietary balance and the desire to move better to live better, for a real re-education in wellbeing on an everyday level.

Divine treatments, two- or four-hand massages under jets of lukewarm spring water (like the indescribable Vichy shower at the Les Célestins spa) or specialised spa programs, from the 'office aches' special at Cambo-les-Bains to the Poids plume (Featherweight) program at Michel Guérard's weight-loss village at Eugénie-les-Bains … A few examples of the wellspring of creativity!

1200 springs
France lays claim to 20% of Europe's registered springs.

A world first:
scientific studies demonstrate the beneficial effects of spa cures, not only for rheumatism conditions but also in the area of obesity, dermatology and anxiety.
In order to better assess the 'delivered health benefit' of a form of treatment that offers relief to half a million French people (and their prescriptions) every year … a battery of scientific studies is under way.

Fresh start
A thermal plankton with unique healing powers is working wonders at Molitg-les-Bains.

Thalassotherapy
marine forces

The riches of the ocean have produced a wave sweeping the coasts and offering a wide range of specialised treatments for relaxation and total fitness!

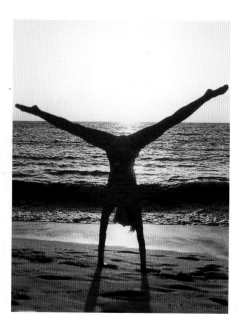

LIFE DOESN'T LACK SALT

Sea water is an absolute marvel that concentrates mineral salts, trace elements (iodine, calcium, magnesium), proteins, plankton, algae and ocean clays. Reason enough to have a dip! Which is what thalassotherapy provides, by offering an iodised cocktail with all of the benefits of the ocean, under medical supervision. At the same time it fills our lungs with **very pure air, charged with ultra-invigorating ozone and negative ions,** which whip up the blood and strengthen the defences.

Drawn from the open sea away from the coast (it's safer), the sea water is heated to 34°C so that it penetrates the pores of the skin better and takes care of every little (and large) need of our bodies, which are exhausted by every kind of pollution and stress. Baths, water-jets, showers … Remineralisation, invigoration, elimination of toxins by stimulating the defences of the vital functions … and regeneration as never before.

THALASSOTONIC!

Thalassotherapy includes wraps, pressure therapy, hydrojets and new-wave approaches, traditional treatments combined with sports programs or treatment programs based on alternative medicines (osteopathy, aromatherapy, naturopathy) or Eastern medicines. Depending on your aim and priorities, anything is possible. Since its pioneering days in Roscoff a century ago and Quiberon, there have been innovations in all directions, such as submerged fitness apparatus (Carnac) or dance-thalasso options (Bénodet).

THE WORD FROM THE EXPERT

The primordial milieu of the ocean is infinite in riches with a wealth of promise … realised in the form of a large number of medications. From the prostaglandin found in corals to the multiple uses of cephalosporins, the first antibiotics to come from the sea … To the anticarcinogens discovered in shark stomach and sea sponges!

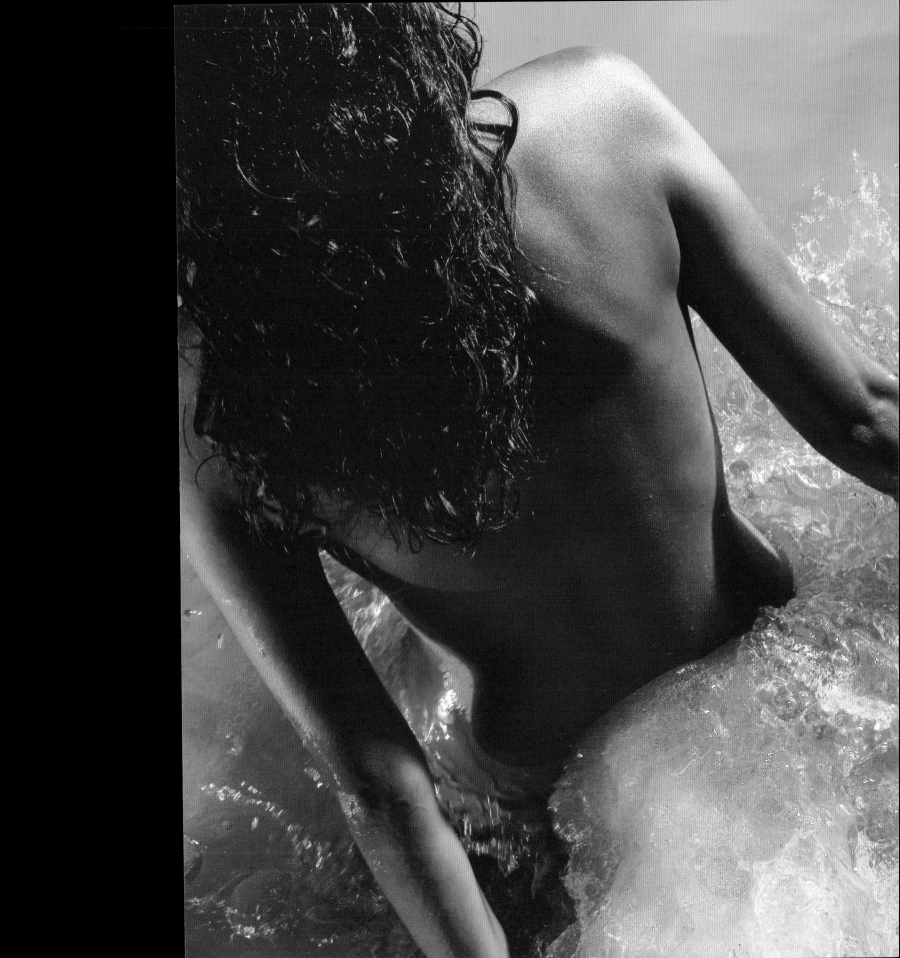

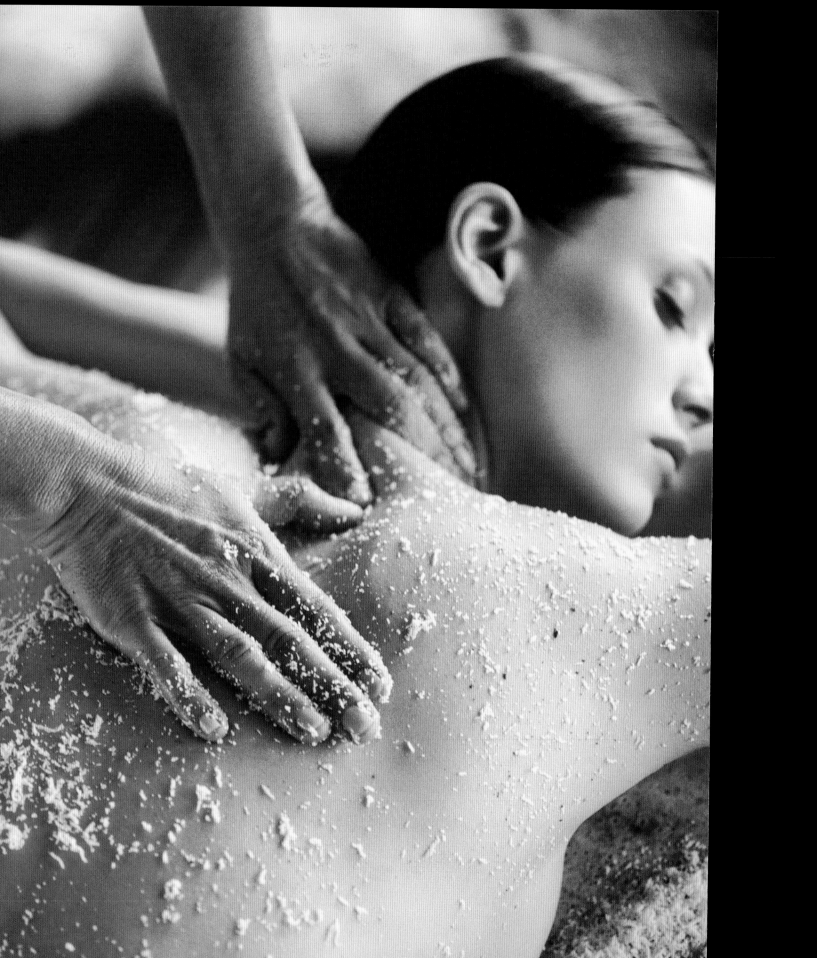

Spa passion

The day spa, apart from being a fashion, is a state of mind. An absolute beauty bubble, disconnected from everyday contingencies. On the other side of the world or in my bathroom, wellbeing is the priority.

SALT AND GINGER, AN EXQUISITE COCKTAIL

… for an exfoliating session that you won't want to scrub from your memory or spectacular plant-based body wraps that earn their laurels: two examples of the imagination at work in spa treatments. Hot stones or spicy delights, wonderful oils or water from the Dead Sea (180 g salt per litre, the absolute record) offering a concentration of minerals and trace elements that is just as staggering, all have their competing sublime recipes, adapting local resources to turn us into worthy descendants of Cleopatra.

A SPA TA-DA!

A name derived from a very lively Belgian spring town in the Ardennes region, popularised in the United States (where it meant simply 'jacuzzi'), before becoming synonymous with beauty breaks of a decidedly luxurious kind. Luxury hotels the world over have followed in the footsteps of Claude Renaudin and Patrick Ribes, who invented the concept for Givenchy in 1985. The idea, to offer exclusive treatments in exceptional settings, is today spread out over five locations (Cheval Blanc and Martinez in France, but also in Canada, Dubai and Mauritius) where, apart from the house treatments (including the No Complex range), there are adaptations of ancient beauty regimes gathered from all over the world by Claude Renaudin, who for example adapted the Hawaiian lomi-lomi (loving touch) after meeting an 80-year-old Hawaiian who invented it, and uses authentic Arizona pebbles for his Canyon Love Therapy.

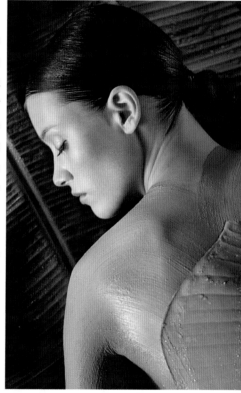

Grand Canyon therapy
The incredible properties of Arizona stones were discovered by a therapist who treated her own sprained ankle after falling down a canyon.

Essential . precious oils

Essential oils are what make aromatherapy one of the most refined forms of therapy. A journey for the nose and the rest of the senses, inhale with abandon.

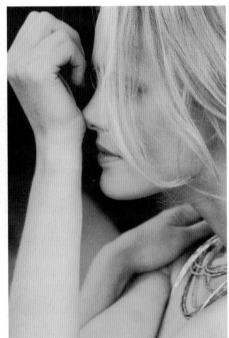

BREATHING IN GOOD HEALTH?

From insomnia to hay fever via skin problems, there are countless applications of aromatherapy, **a perfumed version of phytotherapy** (plant therapy).

Containing no glycerides (unlike their vegetable cousins, they don't stain), essential oils are steam-extracted using a sophisticated and wildly extravagant process. Awe-inspired references are often made to the **five tonnes of petals needed to make a single litre of essence of rose**!

40 ESSENTIAL REASONS to immerse yourself in pleasure

Whether you imbue yourself with fragrances magnified by the warmth of the **bath** or a **massage** (mixed with sweet almond oil, for example), or else via a **fragrance diffuser**, the aromas of the forty-odd recorded essential oils are beneficial for the soul as well as the body. But like any active ingredient, they need to be used in an informed way, in the appropriate dose ... and not left in reach of young children.

No therapeutic trial has confirmed the effectiveness of aromatherapy. However, a recent scientific article demonstrated the effects of perfume on skin immunity: an allergic reaction was able to be controlled using the simple inhalation of a fragrance.

THE STAR CAST OF OILS...

Cypress, borage, evening primrose for improving circulation.

Coriander, mint or nutmeg for stimulation.

Eucalyptus or cinnamon for killing germs.

Cumin and mint for assisting digestion.

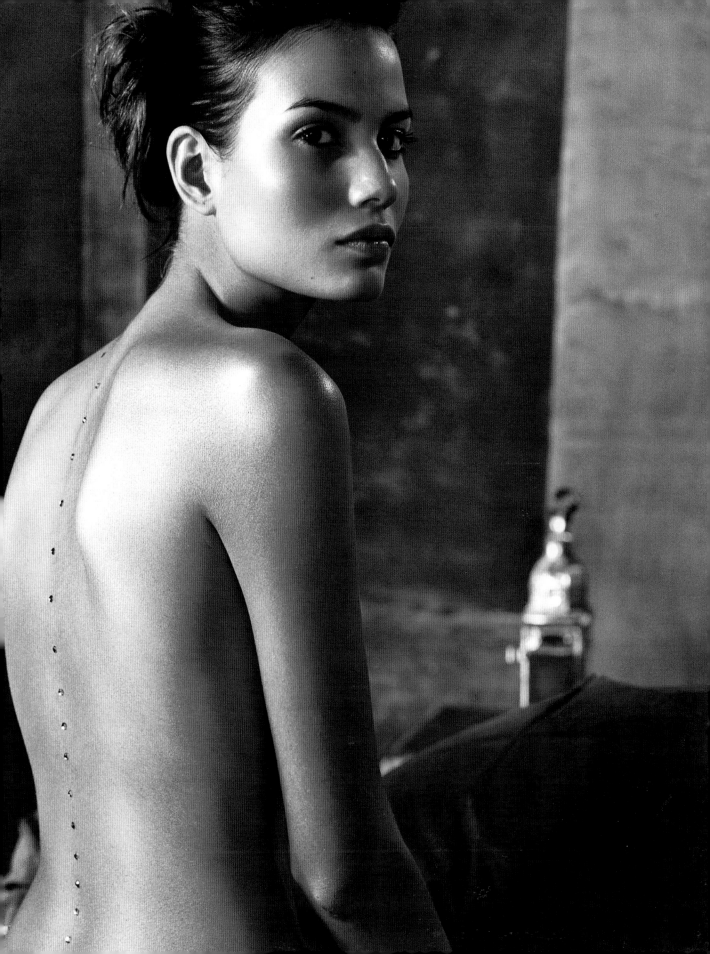

Credits

PHOTOGRAPHER CREDITS

Jean-Claude Amiel (p. 119); **Hugh Arnold** (p. 52, 126); **Aloïs Beer** (p. 94); **Pierre Berdoy** (p. 99); **Bruno Bisang** (p. 18b); **Frederico Cimatti** (p. 121); **Greg Conraux** (p. 4a); **Laurent Darmon** (p. 56, 145, 177, 188, 189, 191); **Patrick Demarchelier** (p. 18c); **Eric Deniset** (p. 22, 40c); **Bruno Fabbris** (p. 130); **Frédéric Farré** (p. 72, 100); **Hans Feurer** (p. 7c); **Christian Giesen** (p. 7b, 62, 63, 82, 151, 190); **Guillaume Girardot** (p. 6i, 11, 18a, 49, 71b, 116, 167, 182, 186); **Frédéric Gresse** (p. 163); **Emmanuelle Hauguel** (p. 44, 51, 131); **Bertrand Jacquot** (p. 59, 60, 158a, 168, 169, 170, 171, 172, 173, 174, 175); **Jean-François Jonvelle** (p. 6e, 6h, 68, 89); **Bruno Juminer** (p. 13, 97, 108); **Sylvie Lancrenon** (p. 154, 155, 158b, 159, 161); **François Lange** (p. 7g, 40a); **LIERAC** (p. 4b, 5a, 9, 134, 136, 137, 138, 139, 140, 141); **Alain Longeaud** (p. 95); **Jeff Manzetti** (p. 21, 35, 50, 58, 64, 93, 187); **Stéphane Martinelli** (p. 6f, 7f, 181, 184); **Matthias** (p. 96b); **MIXA** (p. 75, 77, 78, 80, 81); **Michel Momy** (p. 25); **Marc Montezin** (p. 6a, 43, 48, 84, 85, 180, 183); **Pascal Moraiz** (p. 96a); **Marc Neuhoff** (p. 147); **Pierre Nicou** (p. 90); **Marc Philbert** (p. 47, 111); **Bruno Poinsard** (p. 5b, 6k, 31, 55, 86, 104, 112, 129); **André Rau** (p. 14); **Patrice Reumont** (p. 6c, 71a, 107, 164, 165, 166); **Martin Rusch** (p. 152); **Pierre Sabatier** (p. 27, 96c); **Christian Sauter** (p. 7h); **Lothar Schmid** (p. 6j, 7i, 29, 39, 40b, 122); **Kristian Schuller** (p. 6g); **Manfred Seelow** (p. 117); **Jens Stuart** (p. 156, 157); **Jérôme Tisné** (p. 6d); **Cees Van Gelderen** (p. 6b, 36, 66, 67, 69, 115, 149, 179); **Sabine Vuilliard** (p. 7d, 142); **Alexandre Weinberger** (couverture, p. 17); **Kenneth Willardt** (p. 18d, 32a, 32b, 71c, 71d); **Michael Wirth** (p. 125).

MODEL CREDITS

Crystal Stecci Sellan (p. 40a, 84); **Dominique Models** Sarah Marivoet (p. 172, 173, 174, 175); **Elite** Holte Bettina (p. 154, 155, 159, 161), Suzanna (p. 72); **Ford** Dari (p. 21), Davina (p. 25); **IMG** Karin Anderson (p. 40b, 107, 164, 165, 166), Olga Maliouk (p. 100), Karin Astrid (p. 142), Frida (p. 158a, 168, 169, 170, 171), Ivana (p. 59, 60), Marina (p. 149); **Marilyn** Tatiana Ruban (p. 152); **Metropolitan** Askevolde Janicke (p. 145), Jarnie (p. 17), Sanda (p. 66, 67, 115); **Next** Anja Rubick (p. 32a); Anne Flore (p. 64), Camilla Thorsend (p. 56, 188, 189), Daniela Kanter (p. 18d), Emma Hemming (p. 68, 89), Juliane Martins (p. 51), Pania Rose (p. 29, 122, 131); **Viva** Marie (p. 190); **Women Management** Nieves (p. 129).

FACE AND BODY BY **marie claire**

Editorial Director: Thierry Lamarre.
Concept, interviews and Editing: Josette Milgram.
Layout editing: Nicolas Valoteau.
Assistant editor: Either Studio.
Editorial assistant: Adeline Lobut.
Artwork and design: Domitille Peyron and Sylvie Creusy, assisted by Audrey Lacoudre.
Translation: Kim Allen Gleed

First published in French by
Éditions MARIE CLAIRE in 2008
© 2008, Éditions Marie Claire – Société d'Information et de Créations (SIC)

This edition
Published in 2009 by Murdoch Books Pty Limited

Murdoch Books Australia
Pier 8/9
23 Hickson Road
Millers Point NSW 2000
Phone: +61 (0) 2 8220 2000
Fax: +61 (0) 2 8220 2558
www.murdochbooks.com.au

Murdoch Books UK Limited
Erico House, 6th Floor
93–99 Upper Richmond Road
Putney, London SW15 2TG
Phone: +44 (0) 20 8785 5995
Fax: +44 (0) 20 8785 5985
www.murdochbooks.co.uk

The National Library of Australia Cataloguing-in-Publication Data:

Milgram, Josette.
Marie Claire face & body / Josette Milgram.
ISBN 9781741962062 (pbk.).
Marie Claire fashion and beauty
Includes index.
Skin--Care and hygiene. Beauty, Personal
646.7

Printed by 1010 Printing International Limited in 2009.
PRINTED IN CHINA